THIRD EDITION

BEGIN HAIRDRESSING AND BARBERING

The Official Guide to Level One

THIRD EDITION

BEGIN HAIRDRESSING AND BARBERING

The Official Guide to Level One

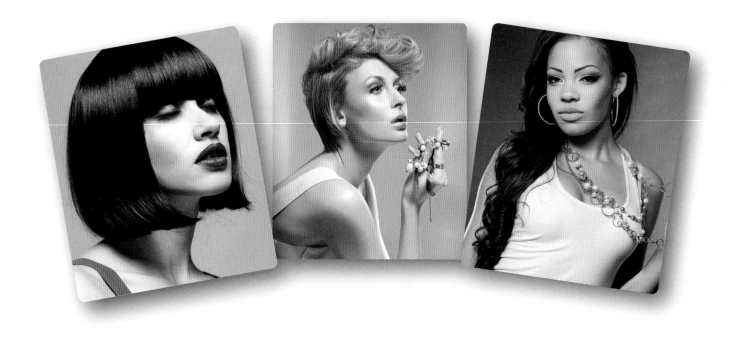

MARTIN GREEN

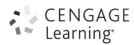

CENGAGE
Learning®

Australia • Brazil • Japan • Korea • Mexico • Singapore • Spain • United Kingdom • United States

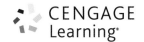

Begin Hairdressing and Barbering – The Official Guide to Level One, Third Edition
Martin Green

Development Editor: Catharine Esmat

Senior Production Editor: Alison Burt

Senior Manufacturing Buyer: Eyvett Davis

Typesetter: MPS Limited

Cover design: HCT Creative

Text design: Design Deluxe

For product information and technology assistance,
contact **emea.info@cengage.com**.

For permission to use material from this text or product,
and for permission queries,
email **emea.permissions@cengage.com**.

British Library Cataloguing-in-Publication Data
A catalogue record for this book is available from the British Library.

ISBN: 978-1-4080-7508-1

Cengage Learning EMEA
Cheriton House, North Way, Andover, Hampshire, SP10 5BE
United Kingdom

Cengage Learning products are represented in Canada by Nelson Education Ltd.

For your lifelong learning solutions, visit **www.cengage.co.uk**

Purchase your next print book, e-book or e-chapter at
www.cengagebrain.com

Printed in China by RR Donnelley
Print Number 01   Print Year 2014

HABIA SERIES LIST

Hairdressing

Student textbooks

Hairdressing and Barbering The Foundations: The Official Guide to Hairdressing and Barbering at Level 2 REVISED 7e *Martin Green*

Hairdressing and Barbering The Foundations: The Official Guide to Hairdressing and Barbering VRQ at Level 2 1e *Martin Green*

Professional Hairdressing and Barbering: The Official Guide to Level 3 7e *Martin Green and Leo Palladino*

The Pocket Guide to Key Terms for Hairdressing *Martin Green*

The Official Guide to the City & Guilds Certificate in Salon Service 1e *John Armstrong with Anita Crosland, Martin Green and Lorraine Nordmann*

The Colour Book: The Official Guide to Colour for NVQ Levels 2 & 3 1e *Tracey Lloyd with Christine McMillan-Bodell*

eXtensions: The Official Guide to Hair Extensions 1e *Theresa Bullock*

Salon Management *Martin Green*

Men's Hairdressing: Traditional and Modern Barbering 3e *Maurice Lister*

African-Caribbean Hairdressing 3e *Sandra Gittens*

The World of Hair Colour 1e *John Gray*

The Cutting Book: The Official Guide to Cutting at S/NVQ Levels 2 and 3 *Jane Goldsbro and Elaine White*

Professional Hairdressing titles

Trevor Sorbie: The Bridal Hair Book 1e *Trevor Sorbie and Jacki Wadeson*

The Art of Dressing Long Hair 1e *Guy Kremer and Jacki Wadeson*

Patrick Cameron: Dressing Long Hair 1e *Patrick Cameron and Jacki Wadeson*

Patrick Cameron: Dressing Long Hair 2 1e *Patrick Cameron and Jacki Wadeson*

Bridal Hair 1e *Pat Dixon and Jacki Wadeson*

Professional Men's Hairdressing: The Art of Cutting and Styling 1e *Guy Kremer and Jacki Wadeson*

Essensuals, the Next Generation Toni and Guy: Step by Step 1e *Sacha Mascolo, Christian Mascolo and Stuart Wesson*

Mahogany Hairdressing: Step to Cutting, Colouring and Finishing Hair 1e *Martin Gannon and Richard Thompson*

Mahogany Hairdressing: Advanced Looks 1e *Martin Gannon and Richard Thompson*

The Total Look: The Style Guide for Hair and Make-up Professional 1e *Ian Mistlin*

Trevor Sorbie: Visions in Hair 1e *Trevor Sorbie, Kris Sorbie and Jacki Wadeson*

The Art of Hair Colouring 1e *David Adams and Jacki Wadeson*

Beauty therapy

Beauty Basics: The Official Guide to Level 1 3e Revised Edition *Lorraine Nordmann*

Beauty Therapy – The Foundations: The Official Guide to Level 2 VRQ 6e *Lorraine Nordmann*

Beauty Therapy – The Foundations: The Official Guide to Level 2 6e *Lorraine Nordmann*

Professional Beauty Therapy – The Official Guide to Level 3 4e Revised Edition *Lorraine Nordmann*

The Pocket Guide to Key Terms for Beauty Therapy *Lorraine Nordmann and Marian Newman*

The Official Guide to the City & Guilds Certificate in Salon Services 1e *John Armstrong with Anita Crosland, Martin Green and Lorraine Nordmann*

The Complete Guide to Make-Up 1e *Suzanne Le Quesne*

The Encyclopedia of Nails 1e *Jacqui Jefford and Anne Swain*

The Art of Nails: A Comprehensive Style Guide to Nail Treatments and Nail Art 1e *Jacqui Jefford*

Nail Artistry 1e *Jacqui Jefford*

The Complete Nail Technician 3e *Marian Newman*

Manicure, Pedicure and Advanced Nail Techniques 1e *Elaine Almond*

The Official Guide to Body Massage 2e *Adele O'Keefe*

An Holistic Guide to Massage 1e *Tina Parsons*

Indian Head Massage 2e *Muriel Burnham-Airey and Adele O'Keefe*

Aromatherapy for the Beauty Therapist 1e *Valerie Worwood*

An Holistic Guide to Reflexology 1e *Tina Parsons*

An Holistic Guide to Anatomy and Physiology 1e *Tina Parsons*

The Essential Guide to Holistic and Complementary Therapy 1e *Helen Beckmann and Suzanne Le Quesne*

The Spa Book 1e *Jane Crebbin-Bailey, Dr John Harcup, and John Harrington*

SPA: The Official Guide to Spa Therapy at Levels 2 and 3, *Joan Scott and Andrea Harrison*

Nutrition: A Practical Approach 1e *Suzanne Le Quesne*

Hands on Sports Therapy 1e *Keith Ward*

Encyclopedia of Hair Removal: A Complete Reference to Methods, Techniques and Career Opportunities, *Gill Morris and Janice Brown*

The Anatomy and Physiology Workbook: For Beauty and Holistic Therapies Levels 1–3. *Tina Parsons*

The Anatomy and Physiology CD-Rom

Beautiful Selling: The Complete Guide to Sales Success in the Salon *Rath Langley*

The Official Guide to the Diploma in Hair and Beauty Studies at Foundation Level 1e *Jane Goldsbro and Elaine White*

The Official Guide to the Diploma in Hair and Beauty Studies at Higher Level 1e *Jane Goldsbro and Elaine White*

The Official Guide to Foundation Learning in Hair and Beauty 1e *Jane Goldsbro and Elaine White*

Contents

PART ONE The Workplace

PART TWO **Practical Skills**

Foreword by Habia

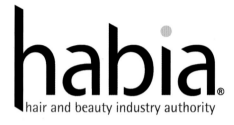

What can one say about Martin Green that has not already been said in these forewords? Martin has dedicated his life to developing learners. Always at the forefront of technology and didactic learning, Martin demonstrates once again his range of skills and depth of knowledge of the hairdressing industry.

If you spend some time perusing these pages, you'll see why Martin is still producing great books that are ever popular with learners in this profession.

If you want to rise to the top of the hairdressing industry, I urge you to invest in this superb study guide. As Director of Standards and Qualifications for Habia, I'm delighted that this book reflects the current standards and ethos of Habia.

Jane Goldsbro
Director of Standards and Qualifications
Habia

About Habia

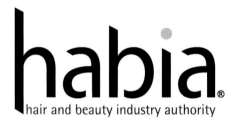

Habia, the Hair and Beauty Industry Authority, is appointed by government to represent employers in the hair and beauty sector. Habia's main role is to manage the development of the National Occupational Standards (NOS) for hairdressing, barbering, beauty therapy, nails and spa. They are developed by industry for industry and represent best practice when achieving skills and knowledge for a particular job role.

Habia is also responsible for the development and implementation of apprenticeship frameworks and for issuing apprenticeship certificates, alongside providing information to employers on government initiatives that may affect the hair and beauty industry – be it educational, environmental or financial. A central point of contact for information, Habia provides guidance on careers, business development, legislation, salon health and safety. Habia is part of SkillsActive, the Sector Skills Council that covers hair and beauty, sports and the active leisure sector.

About VTCT

VTCT is a lead specialist awarding organization in the hair and beauty sectors offering a varied suite of qualifications to suit all needs and abilities. With 50 years of experience, VTCT has a full qualification package covering the following additional sectors: Sport and Active Leisure, Hospitality and Catering, Complementary Therapies and Business and Retail.

VTCT offers qualifications to over 700 colleges and training providers both in the UK and internationally, with centres as far away as India, South Africa and Australia as well as many throughout Europe.

www.vtct.org.uk

About the author

Martin Green is a highly experienced hairdressing practitioner and college lecturer with over 40 years' experience in the industry. During that time, he has been a consultant for Habia where he was part of the original team that created the first industry standards. He has worked for awarding authorities such as the City and Guilds of London Institute, where he was a regional verifier for the south west, and at the Vocational Training Charitable Trust where he wrote a wide range of assessment materials.

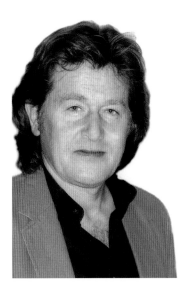

Martin is author of the *Official Guides to Hairdressing*. These include *Begin Hairdressing Level 1*, *Hairdressing and Barbering Level 2* and *Professional Hairdressing Level 3*. All are bestsellers in their domain.

Martin's energy and passion for his craft are keenly demonstrated through his being a unique blend of practitioner, teacher and author. His enthusiasm has been unyielding and he has shown a deep commitment to the development of e-learning and online resources as well as print materials.

Martin has won a national JISC Hi5 award for developing e-learning at advanced level in the *Widening Participation in Education* category, in recognition of his achievements in this sector.

Acknowledgements

The author and publisher would like to thank the following contributors who have collaborated so closely with us to produce this book.

For constant partnership in reflecting industry standards:

Habia

VTCT

For expert review and feedback on the material:

Lesley Elliott of Lincoln College

Peter Health of Waltham College

Sheridan Drew of South Devon College

For providing images:

BaByliss PRO

Balmain Hair

Banbury Postiche Ltd

Beauty Express

Cinderella Hair

Connect-2-Hair Ltd

Denman

Dr Seymour Weaver

E. A. Ellison & Co Ltd

Glove Club

Goldwell

Habia

Hair Tools Limited

HMSO

HSE

iStockphoto

King Research Inc

L'Oréal Professionnel

Montibel.lo Product Images

Patrick Cameron

REM UK (Ltd)

Saks Hair & Beauty

Shutterstock

The Real Shave Company

Theresa Bullock

Wahl (UK) Ltd

Wella

The publisher would like to thank the many copyright holders who have generously granted us permission to reproduce material throughout this textbook. Every effort has been made to contact all rights holders, but in the unlikely event that anything has been overlooked please contact the publisher directly and we will happily make the necessary arrangements at the earliest opportunity.

For their help with the photoshoots:

Staff and Organizers at Andover College

Louise Holm

Claire Napoli

Ken Franklin

Nathan Allan

Sita Gill

Justin Lawrence-Smith

Jenny Noakes

Pauline Reynolds

Jo Harris

Debra Rowbotham

Shelley Rider

Credit list

Babyliss Pro – 36 tl1, 36 tl2, 37 mr; **Balmain UK** – 160 tl, 160 bl; **Banbury Postiche Ltd** – 43 ml1, 43 ml2, 43 bl, 44 tl1, 44 tl2; **Barbicide** – 67 br; **Beuaty Express** – 63 br; **Cengage Learning** – 114 tl1, 114 tl2, 126 bl1, 126 bl2, 127 ml1, 127 bl1, 127 bl2, 130 tl, 130 bl, 130 br, 143 ml, 143 mr, 147 tl, 155 tl1, 155 tm1, 155 tr1, 155 tl2, 155 tm2, 155 tr2, 155 bl, 155 bm, 155 br, 156 tl, 156 tm, 156 tr, 156 bl, 156 bm, 156 br; **Cinderella Hair www.cinderellahair.co.uk** – 162 bl; **CONNECT-2-HAIR** – 164 tl; **Denman** – 22 bl, 23 tr, 24 tl1, 29 ml, 33 tr2; **Dr Seymour Weaver** – 150 bl; **E A Ellison & Co Ltd** – 18 tl3, 19 tr, 20 tl1, 21 tr1, 25 mr, 26 tm1, 28 tl, 30 tl1, 31 ml, 31 mr, 42 tl, 59 bl, 67 tr2; **Goldwell** – 149 tr; **Goldwell UK** – 47 bm; **Hair Tools Ltd** – 34 tl1, 35 tr, 35 bl, 35 br; **HairTools** – 187 bl; **HMSO** – 62 bl, 62 br; **HSE** – 64 ml; **iStockphoto** – 67 tr1 (© KevinDyer), 73 ml, 81 bl, 127 ml2 (© diane39), 141 bl (© Konstantynov), 148 br (© RuslanDashinsky), 190 bl (© herkisi), 192 tl (© onebluelight), 199 tr (© pfrank1978), 202 tl (© DIGIcal), 204 bm (© alwekelo); **Kent** – 26 tm2; **L'Oréal Professionnel** – 48 tl; **Nathan Allan Photography** – 114 bl, 115 tl1, 115 tm1, 115 tr1, 115 tl2, 115 tm2, 115 tr2, 115 tl3, 115 tm3, 115 tr3, 115 tl4, 115 tm4, 115 tr4, 118 tl1, 118 tm1, 118 tr1, 118 tl2, 118 tm2, 118 tr2, 132 tl1, 132 tm1, 132 tr1, 132 bl1, 132 bl2, 132 br2, 133 tl, 133 tm1, 133 tr, 133 bl, 133 bm, 133 br, 135 tl, 135 tr, 135 ml, 135 mr1, 135 bl, 135 br, 145 tl, 145 tr, 145 ml, 145 mr, 145 bl, 145 br, 147 bl1, 147 bm1, 147 br1, 147 bl2, 147 bm2, 147 br2, 151 bl1, 151 bm1, 151 br1, 151 bl2, 151 bm2, 151 br2, 153 bl1, 153 br1, 153 bl2, 153 br2, 153 bl3, 153 br3, 154 tl1, 154 tm1, 154 tr1, 154 tl2, 154 tm2, 154 tr2, 154 bl, 154 bm, 154 br, 169 tl, 169 tm, 169 tr, 169 bl, 169 bm, 169 br, 175 tl, 175 tm, 175 tr, 179 bl1, 179 bm1, 179 br1, 179 bl2, 179 bm2, 179 br2, 180 tl1, 180 tm1, 180 tr1, 180 tl2, 180 tm2, 180 tr2, 181 tl1, 181 tm1, 181 tr1, 181 tl2, 181 tm2, 181 tr2, 191 tl1, 191 tm1, 191 tr1, 191 tl2, 191 tm2, 191 tr2, 191 tl3, 191 tm3, 191 tr3, 206 tl1, 206 tm1, 206 tr1, 206 tl2, 206 tm2, 206 tr2; **Ossie Rizzo** – 170 tl, 170 tm, 170 tr, 170 bl, 170 bm, 170 br, 170 bl; **Patrick Cameron** – 22 tl1; **REM UK Ltd** – 69 bl; **Saks Hair and Beauty, www.saks.co.uk** – 87 bl; **Shutterstock** – 2 tl (© Oleg Gekman), 3 tr1 (© Paul Hakimata Photography), 3 tr2 (© Mayer George), 3 tr3 (© YuriyZhuravov), 4 tl1 (© Iancu Cristian), 6 tl (© Petrenko Andriy), 6 bl (© Dmitry Kalinovsky), 8 bl (© wavebreakmedia), 10 ml (© karamysh), 11 tl1 (© Tyler Olson), 11 tl2 (© dean bertoncelj), 11 tl3 (© xjrshimada), 11 bl1 (© Alfred Wekelo), 14 tl1 (© Subbotina Anna), 14 tl2 (© bikeriderlondon), 14 tl3 (© bikeriderlondon), 15 br (© Ikonoklast Fotografie), 16 tl1 (© Valua Vitaly), 27 bm (© YuriyZhuravov), 32 tl (© Rob Bouwman), 33 tr1 (© Rob Byron), 49 bl (© ariadna de raadt), 50 ml (© Gemenacom), 51 ml (© Gemenacom), 53 br (© Monkey Business Images), 54 mr (© Rade Kovac), 56 tr (© margo_black), 58 ml (© Rob Byron), 60 tl (© bikeriderlondon), 61 bl (© bikeriderlondon), 74 br (dean bertoncelj), 76 tr (© Olga Ekaterincheva), 78 tl (© In Green), 79 br (© Tyler Olson), 80 bl (© Tyler Olson), 81 tl, 82 tl (© Viktoria Gavrilina), 85 bl (© Paul Vasarhelyi), 92 tr (© Nadya Korobkova), 94 tl (© ariadna de raadt), 96 ml (© Monkey Business Images), 97 br (© bikeriderlondon), 98 tl (© bikeriderlondon), 98 bl (© bikeriderlondon), 104 tc (© FlexDreams), 105 tl (© Valua Vitaly), 105 tm (© Violanda), 105 tr (© Maksim Toome), 106 tr (© Valua Vitaly), 108 mr (© Inga Ivanova), 110 tl (© Inga Ivanova), 111 mr (© nito),

Introduction by the author

If you are wondering about a career in hairdressing or barbering, then look no further. Here is everything you need to know – all in one place. If you have any doubts about whether this industry is for you, then why not spend some time finding out, while you grow in skill *and* confidence and gain a qualification at the same time.

If you can answer **yes** to most or all of the following questions, then you have come to the right place:

◆ Do you like meeting people and socializing?

◆ Do current fashions and the media motivate you?

◆ Do you aspire to being recognized as a trained professional?

◆ Do you want to gain the respect of other people?

◆ Would you like a career that puts you in control of your own future?

◆ Do you like the idea of making other people feel good about themselves?

◆ Are you creative and good with your hands?

If so, welcome to the fascinating world of hairdressing. All you have to do now is find somewhere to learn and enjoy your training.

Good luck — I wish you every success for the future.

Martin Green

Level 1 in Hairdressing and Barbering

The Level 1 qualification provides the main industry-recognized qualification for salon apprenticeships and college-based courses. The structure of the Level 1 qualification requires the learner to complete a core set of mandatory units, and then make choices for a range of mix and match topics based upon your own particular interests.

NOS: an introduction to standards

Habia, the Hair and Beauty Industry Authority, is the representative organization responsible for defining the standards for our hair and beauty industry. The National Occupational Standards (NOS) that it produces are taken and used by awarding organizations such as City & Guilds (C&G), VTCT or ITEC to create the qualifications that you take part in. Therefore, in simple terms, Habia produces the standards that you work towards and ITEC/C&G/VTCT define the conditions and specifications against which you are assessed.

The NOS used in hairdressing or barbering have a common structure and design. Some of the units are specific to the industry – such as blow-drying, shampooing and conditioning – whereas others such as health and safety or personal effectiveness are common across many vocational sectors. This common structure enables students to be credited with units of competence that are accepted in other industries too. In the past, this has always been a problem, as someone who qualified in one sector was not necessarily acknowledged as being competent in another, even though they had the training and experience.

Level 1 in Hairdressing and Barbering

The mandatory units are:

Unit:
Ensure responsibility for actions to reduce risks to health and safety
Contribute to the development of effective working relationships
Shampoo and condition hair
Prepare for hair services and maintain work areas

The optional units are:

Unit:
Assist with salon reception duties
Blow dry hair
Assist with hair colouring services
Assist with perming hair services
Plait and twist hair using basis techniques
Remove hair extensions
Assist with shaving services

Units and learning outcomes

A unit relates to a specific task or skill area of work. It is the smallest part of a qualification and carries its own credit value, which you can build up to achieve a qualification.

A learning outcome describes in detail the skill and knowledge components of the unit that need to be completed.

For each unit, when all the outcomes have been achieved, a unit certification may be awarded. A Level 1 qualification is made up of a specific number of units required for the occupational area. Some of the units are mandatory (compulsory) and some are optional (not compulsory). All mandatory units must be achieved to gain the Level 1 qualification and a specified number of optional units must be selected to study in addition to the mandatory units to attain the qualification.

Unit title and learning outcomes (example Health and Safety Unit):

Unit title	Learning outcomes
Make sure your own actions reduce risks to health and safety	Identify the hazards and evaluate the risks in your workplace
	Reduce the risks to health and safety in your workplace

The NOS covers the learning outcomes in detail. They specify how each task is to be performed by listing the performance criteria. They also cover the circumstances, conditions or situations in which these actions must be carried out. This is referred to as the range.

Performance criteria

The performance criteria are a list of essential actions. Although these may not necessarily appear in the order in which they should be done, they do provide a definitive checklist of what needs doing. During assessment, these performance criteria form the framework of how a task must be carried out.

Performance criteria
The performance criteria say what you have to do:
1   Communicate with clients in a manner which promotes goodwill, trust and maintains confidentiality.
2   Handle client belongings with care and return them when required.
3   Promptly refer any client concerns to the relevant person.
4   Maintain client comfort and care to the satisfaction of the client.
5   Meet your salon's standards for appearance and behaviour.

Range

The range statements provide a number of conditions or applications in which the learning outcomes must be performed. Quite simply, they state under what particular circumstances, and on what occasions, or in which special situations the activity must take place.

Example range statements identify which situations or circumstances need to be included when carrying out a task. For example:

Range
The range says what you must cover:
1   Actively participate in training and development activities.
2   Actively participate in salon activities.
3   Observe and learn about technical activities.

Essential knowledge underpinning the activity

When you do your work properly, you need to know **why** you are performing your tasks. The terms 'theory', 'learning' and 'principles' generally refer to essential knowledge and understanding, in other words what you **must** know.

Essential knowledge and understanding

The knowledge and understanding tells us what we need to know:

1   How to communicate in a clear, polite, confident way and why this is important.

2   The questioning and listening skills you need in order to find out information.

3   The rules and procedures regarding the methods of communication you use.

4   How to recognize when a client is angry and when a client is confused.

At the point where a task's performance criteria and range have been covered and knowledge has been learnt and understood, we can say that the task has been carried out competently and a skill has been acquired.

Shared knowledge

Units and learning outcomes often share similar components. Therefore some performance criteria used to achieve an outcome from one task are often similar to those required for another. For example:

◆   Maintain effective and safe methods of working when assisting with colouring services

◆   Maintain effective and safe methods of working when assisting with perming services

In this case the knowledge that is essential and underpinning one learning outcome occurs in another. This duplication may at first seem unnecessary, but it is important because of the modular, stand-alone design of the units.

This can be useful in terms of speeding up the learning process as knowledge or skills learnt in one activity are then directly applicable to other tasks. This is also useful when it comes to recording these learnt experiences, because knowledge gained in one situation can be quickly cross-referenced to other similar activities in your portfolio.

Under assessment

Your competence, your ability to carry out a task to a required standard, is judged during assessment. Your ability to carry out the task's 'performance evidence' is observed and checked against the performance criteria. Therefore, your assessor will be watching to see how you carry out your work.

Sometimes it is not possible to cover all the situations that might crop up in one performance. In this case your assessor might ask you questions about what you have done and how you might apply that in different circumstances. To help you get used to this, the activities that appear throughout the book contain many of the types of questions that you might be asked.

Your understanding and background knowledge of work tasks is also measured through questions asked by your assessor. Sometimes you might be asked to give a personal account of what you have learned. This could take the form of writing a sequence of events that need to be done to complete the task satisfactorily. Other questions may ask you about particular tasks; more often than not, these types of questions take the form of short-answer or multiple-choice questions. The activities featured in this book give plenty of examples and opportunities to practise.

About the website

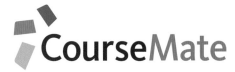

CourseMate is the online interactive partner resource to Cengage Learning publications.

Using our Hairdressing and Barbering Level 1 CourseMate alongside this textbook will provide a richly blended solution to your learning.

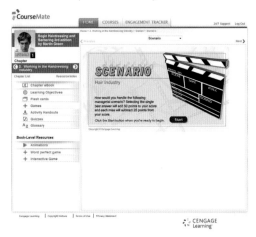

CourseMate is a highly interactive resource which brings course concepts to life. It is designed to support students and lecturers by providing a range of online resources, activities and video footage that perfectly integrate with classroom learning to fulfil the guided learning requirements for each unit.

For students:

◆ Searchable eBook makes finding the right information quick and easy.

◆ Step-by-step videos show you how the professionals carry out key hairdressing techniques.

◆ Interactive multi-choice quizzes enable you to test your knowledge and prepare for assessments.

◆ Online activities and games bring a new dimension to your learning and make it fun.

For lecturers:

◆ Lesson plans at your fingertips ensure you cover the full syllabus.

◆ PowerPoint slides provide easy classroom presentations.

◆ Activity hand-outs are great for students to complete in class or in their own time.

◆ Engagement Tracker tools help you track the progress of each student and monitor their learning.

For further information about CourseMate, please contact **emea.fesales@cengage.com**

About this book

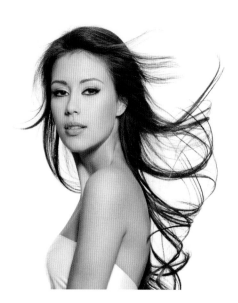

Welcome to the latest edition of the Begin Hairdressing and Barbering series for Level 1 – the perfect learning companion for your Level 1 studies no matter which awarding body qualification you are studying towards.

Updated to reflect the very latest national occupational standards put in place by Habia in 2014, we have reworked this manual to provide:

◆ the quickest and easiest navigation to the services and practices you want to find out about

◆ a comprehensive guide to all aspects of the Level 1 qualification to help prepare you for a career in hairdressing and barbering

◆ a chapter structure that mirrors the latest standards in unit and outcome format

◆ a special double-page layout that makes learning and teaching as intuitive as possible

◆ a detailed glossary and index to help you find terminology and understand key information.

All these features and illustrations have been redesigned and reorganized in order to help you accelerate through your Level 1 programme.

How to use this book

You can use this book in a number of ways. For example:

◆ Study the revised chapter structure and page layouts, which focus on clearly-signposted discrete topics, to cover the key information needed for your training.

◆ Use the book as a quick reference or overview of all aspects of your learning – both theory and practice.

◆ Use the book as a stand-alone course guide covering the A–Z of hairdressing and barbering services at Level 1.

◆ Dip into the book at random and discover the range of topics that are featured, from health and safety, to salon practices, to career development advice.

Our new format with its easy page navigation will help you get the very best from this book. Each chapter opens with a quick look at what you are going to learn, and then extends to cover each element of the programme at the correct level of detail. To help you revise, we include learning summaries and revision questions too.

Pedagogy features

We have designed this book to feature clear signposts throughout, so you know exactly what you are studying no matter which page you are looking at. Browse through the pages and discover the range of topics you are going to learn about while working towards your Level 1 qualification.

The pedagogy features below draw your attention to specific pieces of advice and topic-related activities. Use them to consolidate your learning throughout the book.

HEALTH & SAFETY

These draw your attention to relevant health and safety information throughout the course: an essential aspect of gaining technical skills and practising them correctly.

BEST PRACTICE

Learn how the professionals do it: get the latest advice for fine-tuning your skills, retaining new information and developing your career.

ACTIVITY

These feature within all chapters and provide you with additional tasks to help you further your understanding. All contribute towards your portfolio.

TOP TIP

Share the author's experience and get the benefit of positive suggestions to help you extend your knowledge and skills.

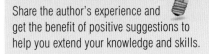

These arrows point you to other sections of the book which explore similar or related topics to ensure a coherent approach to your learning.

At the end of each chapter in this book, you will find an extra page which lists the key learning activities covered in that chapter (with the exception of Chapter 1) and provides an opportunity for revision.

SUMMARY

Summary boxes are found at the end of each chapter. They are designed to help you with the following:

✓ Provide a final reflection on what you have covered within the chapter.

✓ Provide a clearer picture of all the essential aspects of the topics covered, including the tools and equipment you should be using.

✓ Ensure you have a basic understanding of the key principles governing your work.

✓ Ensure you have grasped the necessary health and safety policies that need to be adhered to in your workplace.

REVISION QUESTIONS

Revision sections are found at the end of each chapter. They are designed to help you with the following:

◆ Test your knowledge and understanding of the content of that chapter.

◆ Provide you with an opportunity to demonstrate your learning.

◆ Help you prepare for oral and written assessments.

◆ Help you test yourself and carry out a self-assessment.

◆ Show you where you need further guidance.

◆ Contribute towards your learner portfolio.

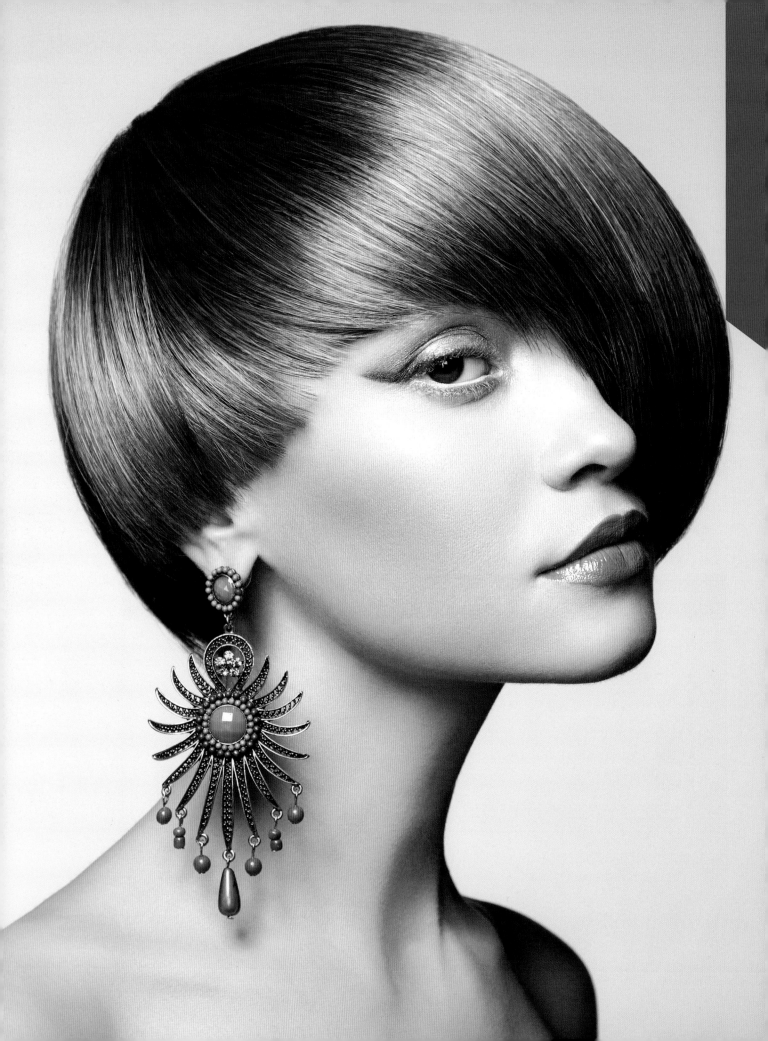

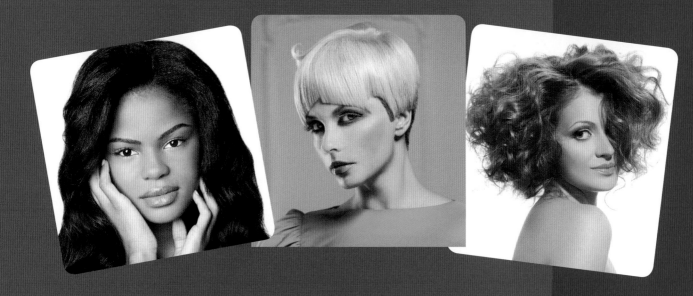

PART ONE

The workplace

Learning to be a professional hairdresser or barber takes more than just being good at cutting, colouring or styling, because our clients want more than just a hair-do.

We must make sure that clients feel welcome from the moment they arrive at the salon in the way that we communicate with them as well as the things that they see and hear in the salon. All of these things should contribute towards helping them to feel relaxed and comfortable throughout their visit, making the whole appointment an enjoyable experience.

In Part One of this book we look at the key customer care aspects of your role, as well as safe working practices, as these are an essential part of the overall service you provide.

1 Introduction to Hairdressing and Barbering

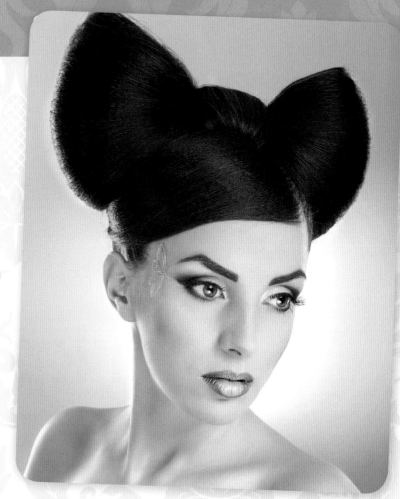

LEARNING OBJECTIVES

When you have finished this chapter you should:

- ◆ know the job roles that people perform within the industry
- ◆ know the working patterns of people working within the sector
- ◆ know the career opportunities available to you in the future
- ◆ understand the services associated with hairdressing and barbering.

KEY TERMS

beard/moustache trimming	cutting	salon-based programme
blow-drying	hair extensions	setting
college-based programme	hair up	shampooing
colour correction	highlights	shaving
colouring	lightening	
conditioning	perming	
consultation	relaxing	

INFORMATION COVERED IN THIS CHAPTER

PRACTICAL SKILLS

Learn about the services associated with barbering

Learn about the services associated with hairdressing

Learn about the jobs that people do within the industry

UNDERPINNING KNOWLEDGE

Know the working hours and patterns of work that people do within the sector

Understand the organizational structure of different size businesses

Know the abbreviations that are used for making appointments for clients

Know what options you have for the future

INTRODUCTION

This is the start of a fulfilling new career for you in an industry that can provide you with many wonderful opportunities. Some of the options open to you when you're qualified are listed here. You could be:

◆ employed and working in a salon or barber's shop

◆ employed and working in an airport or hotel in this country or overseas

◆ self-employed, running your own mobile business

◆ self-employed, running your own barber's shop or salon and employing other staff

◆ taking part in competitions and shows

◆ working in theatre, film or TV.

This chapter will give you a taste of what to expect as you embark on your chosen course. It looks at the work of hairdressers and barbers, the services they provide and typical working patterns for people employed in this sector.

What will I be learning?

Before this question can be answered, we have to look at the different routes or qualifications that are available at Level 1 and also at Levels 2 and 3. The reason we have to look beyond your current Level 1 programme is that, on its own, Level 1 does not qualify you to work as a stylist in a salon. Level 1 qualifies you to help out by assisting other stylists.

TOP TIP

Remember: Level 1 on its own will not get you a job as a stylist; you will need to progress to Level 2 to achieve this.

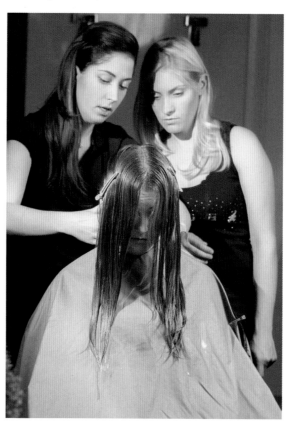

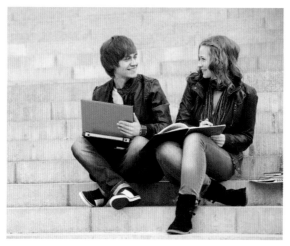

Routes for progressing beyond Level 1

The table opposite provides an overview of the things that are covered in Level 1, together with routes for progression and content for Levels 2 and 3.

Courses available in hairdressing and barbering		
Course level	**Course content/aims**	**On completion, you will be able to:**
Level 1 Hairdressing and barbering	This qualification will enable you to: ✓ Develop your practical hairdressing and barbering skills to a basic level. ✓ Project the professional image needed to work in a personal service industry. ✓ Develop team-working skills, necessary for working with others in a salon. ✓ Identify and reduce risks and hazards associated with health and safety.	Assist in a salon and: ✓ Work on a salon reception. ✓ Have basic skills in dressing and blow-drying hair. ✓ Apply temporary colour. ✓ Shampoo and condition hair. ✓ Display retail stock. ✓ Plait and twist hair. ✓ Style men's hair. ✓ Promote products and services to clients. ✓ Provide scalp massage.
Level 2 Hairdressing and barbering	This qualification will enable you to: ✓ Cut women's and men's hair. ✓ Style, dress and finish women's and men's hair. ✓ Provide consultation services. ✓ Shampoo, condition and treat hair. ✓ Demonstrate good health and safety practices. ✓ Colour and lighten hair. ✓ Perm and neutralize hair. ✓ Provide scalp massage. ✓ Promote services and products. ✓ Display stock effectively. ✓ Work on reception.	Get a job: ✓ Working at a junior stylist level as a women's hairdresser. ✓ Working at a junior stylist level as a men's barber. ✓ Working as a technician in colouring and perming. ✓ Working as a receptionist.
Level 3 Hairdressing and barbering	This qualification will enable you to: ✓ Creatively cut and restyle women's and men's hair. ✓ Creatively style, dress and finish women's and men's hair. ✓ Creatively dress long hair. ✓ Provide advanced consultation services. ✓ Creatively colour and lighten hair. ✓ Carry out colour correction services. ✓ Creatively perm long and short hair. ✓ Help plan promotional events. ✓ Take part in external shows, exhibitions and competitions. ✓ Monitor health and safety practices.	Get a job: ✓ Working at a senior stylist level as a women's hairdresser. ✓ Working at a senior stylist level as a men's barber. ✓ Working as a senior technician in creative colouring and perming. ✓ Doing bridal hair work. ✓ Helping with promotional events and the planning of shows. ✓ Working as a receptionist.

How will I be learning?

Again, it will depend upon which route you take to achieving your qualification. If you choose the **salon-based programme**, you will be learning all of your practical aspects for hairdressing and barbering in the salon (i.e. on the job).

However, hairdressing and barbering are not just about practical activities; there are many other things you need to know in order to do the job properly. Therefore, in addition to practical tasks, you will be learning the theoretical side of the craft such as health and safety and hair science.

The salon where you work may be able to deliver these aspects of the course themselves, but if they are affiliated to a private training provider, then they may operate some other form of delivery, perhaps on a day release basis.

Taking both aspects of the course into consideration, you can expect to be working in a salon at least four days per week and possibly one other day away from the salon on day release. This could be at a local college or at a training centre.

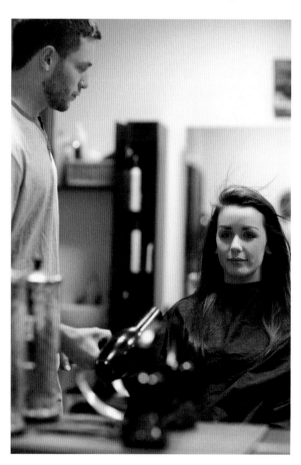

TOP TIP

In order to achieve a qualification, the awarding organization (VTCT, C&G, ITEC) will have provided the college with guidelines on how long the course should take to deliver. For example, Level 2 in hairdressing takes 480 hours of guided learning to achieve (480 GLH).

Take time to discuss your client's requirements both before and during salon services. Once you establish a good rapport with your client, you can build trust and perform at your best.

Course	College-based	Delivery	Salon-based	Delivery	Note
Level 1 hairdressing and barbering 26 weeks	☑	Full-time	NA	NA	
Level 2 hairdressing one-year course	☑	Full-time		Full-time	Only as part of a two-year L3 course
Level 2 hairdressing two-year course	☑	Part-time	☑	Full-time	
Level 2 barbering one-year course	☑	Full-time		Full-time	Only as part of a two-year L3 course
Level 2 barbering two-year course	☑	Part-time	☑	Full-time	
Level 3 hairdressing one-year course	☑	Full-time	NA	NA	
Level 3 hairdressing two-year course	☑	Part-time	☑	Full-time	Standard apprenticeship
Level 3 barbering one-year course	☑	Full-time	NA	NA	
Level 3 barbering two-year course	☑	Part-time	☑	Full-time	Standard apprenticeship

> **TOP TIP**
> Salons and barber shops are not able to offer part-time programmes.

If, on the other hand, you choose the **college-based course**, you will attend college on either a part-time or full-time basis. The pattern of attendance will depend on the type of course applied for, but generally speaking, a college breaks down the number of hours that it takes to learn a qualification level, and then works out how many days are needed to complete this in one academic year.

For example, a course that has 480 hours of learning allocated to it will probably be attended as two-and-a-half days per week for 36 weeks between September and the following July.

> **TOP TIP**
> There are three college terms in the academic year and most courses start in September.

Services within hairdressing and barbering

Hairdressers and barbers provide many services for their clients, and the number is increasing all the time. As a trainee hairdresser or barber, you need to know the range of services that are available in your salon and what processes they involve. You will also need to be familiar with the technical terms used. For example, a cut and blow-dry service involves:

◆ client consultation

◆ shampooing

◆ conditioning

◆ cutting

◆ blow-drying

◆ heat styling.

> For more in-depth information on any of these services, turn to the relevant chapters within this book.

> For more information on communication and appointments, see Chapter 5.

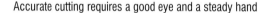

Accurate cutting requires a good eye and a steady hand

When a client books a service, they may be asking for a cut and blow-dry, but they will not know that this will involve several other processes; they would simply assume that the cut and blow-dry is all they need.

As a trainee, you may spend time working in and around reception. When booking appointments you need to know what happens during each service in order to allow the right amount of time for the stylist to provide the client's service properly and thoroughly.

The following table looks at the main services that you need to know and the things they cover. The abbreviations in the table are those that are used in the appointment book.

TOP TIP

Each hairdressing or barbering service has its own abbreviation that is used in the appointment system.

Service name	Abbreviation for appointments book	What happens in this service
Consultation	Cons	A two-way discussion involving the stylist and client to find out their requirements, followed by an examination of their hair/scalp to find any factors/reasons that may affect the planned service/treatment.
Shampooing	**S**/S	A cleansing process that prepares the hair for further services.
Conditioning	Cond or Treat	A process (normally completed after shampooing) that will improve the look, feel, handling and physical properties of the hair.
Blow-drying	B/D	A general term for a method of drying and styling hair by using a variety of round or flat hair brushes to create directional lift and/or volume and/or movement.
Setting	S/**S**	A general term for a method of positioning and fixing various sized rollers in wet or dry hair to create directional lift and/or volume and/or movement.
Cutting	D/C or W/C	A collective name for a variety of techniques and methods that use scissors, thinners, shapers, razors and electric clippers to trim, shape, style and restyle men's and women's hair.
Colouring	Ret or FhCol	A collective name for artificially changing part or all of a client's hair by using temporary, semi-permanent, quasi-permanent or permanent hair colour.
Highlights	H/L	A general term for a partial head colouring process, which may involve lightening or darkening areas of the hair to produce dual tonal or multi tonal effects.
Colour correction	ColCor	A collective name for a variety of colouring techniques and applications, which are used in order to correct an undefined number of artificial colouring problems or mistakes.
Perming	PW	A general term used for permanently changing the properties of hair in order to add volume, movement or curl, or alternatively to change the direction of the natural lie of the hair.
Relaxing	Relax	A general term used for permanently changing the properties of hair in order to reduce natural movement or curl.
Hair up	H/U or P/U	A collective term that covers a wide range of plaiting, curling, folding and positioning techniques, for fixing and dressing longer hair (or extended hair) into a variety of elaborate effects.
Hair extensions	Ext	A general term that covers a wide range of systems and methods for adding artificial or natural hair to a client's existing hair, to add length, density or colour.
Beard/moustache Trimming	Brd Trm	A barbering service for men that involves cutting and styling the facial hair into a variety of managed shapes using scissors, a razor or electric clippers.
Shaving	Shv	A barbering service for men that involves cutting the facial hair using a 'cut-throat' razor and/or electric clippers.

Jobs within the hairdressing industry

The jobs that you do within hairdressing and barbering and the scope for progressing onwards in a job will depend on the size of the business you work in. There are many different types of businesses – from those that are very large and on a global scale to small, independent firms.

Examples of different business models		
Type of business	**How do they operate?**	**How many people do they employ?**
International	A company with outlets on many continents or in many countries	10,000–100,000
Large national chain	A company with many outlets in one country	150–1000
Regional chain	Either a company, sole-trader or partnership with 3–10 salons within a geographical region (i.e. South East)	50–250
Local chain	Either a company, sole-trader or partnership with a couple of salons within a county (i.e. Oxon)	25–50
Independent	Either a company, sole-trader or partnership that has one salon	5–15
Mobile	A sole-trader who visits people in their homes or works from home	one (self)

ACTIVITY

Find out the differences between the following business structures:

1. Company
2. Partnership
3. Sole-trader

Examples of different business entities:

1. *International, e.g. Regis Corporation* – a very large international salon group with 13,000 outlets under many branded salon names such as Supercuts, Sassoon Salon, Regis Salons, MasterCuts and SmartStyle. The Regis Corporation owns many of the salons and the others are run as franchised businesses.

2. *Large, e.g. Headmasters* – an expanding London group with over 40 salons in different parts of the capital.

3. *Regional, e.g. Dimensions* – a county-wide group in the north of England, offering hair and beauty options along with training and education.

4. *Local, e.g. Philosophy* – a small company in the heart of England with a few salons.

5. *Independent* – the vast majority of salons in the UK are run by employers as sole-traders or partnerships, with over 35,000 shops in this category.

Different groups vary considerably in size; as a rule, the larger the salon the more complex the organizational structure. The examples opposite show two very different company structures, one large and one very small.

Large company structure

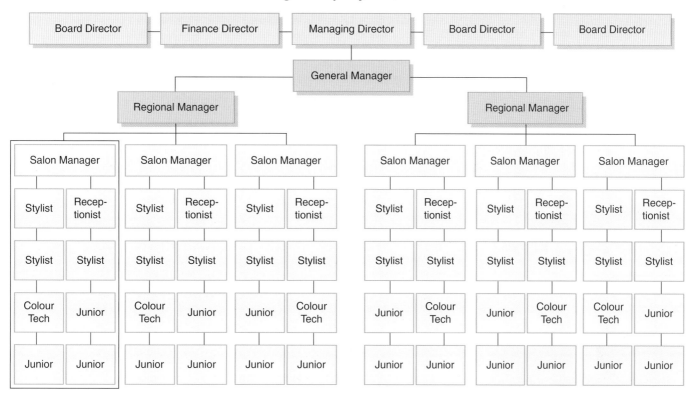

At the lower level of each chart is the junior stylist, who assists qualified staff and carries out some client services. Next up are the hairdressers – they could be stylists or barbers, depending on the salon. Larger salons may have specialist colourists, who carry out all the hair colouring in the salon, and other staff such as a receptionist. Above the hairdressers will be the manager or owner who runs the salon. Large franchises employ regional managers and directors.

As you progress in your career, gaining more experience and qualifications, you will find that your status and salary will change too. If there is a visible route for you to progress within the corporate structure you may find that the package they can offer you (i.e. pension, company car, holiday entitlements, fringe benefits, etc.) makes it worthwhile staying within that structure.

However, sometimes you will find that moving to another salon is the only way that you can progress. Other than that, and with a suitable amount of experience behind you, you may be considering a business venture of your own.

Small independent structure

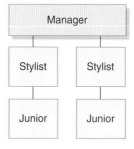

Working time expectations

Whatever you choose to do, you will need to be aware of the implications of working within a personal services industry. Service industries depend on people who are prepared to pay for the services offered – the clients. You need to remember that the client has a life and interests of their own and in order for you to count on them as one of your clients you need to provide a service that they are happy to pay for, at a time that is convenient to them.

In the case of a salon this could mean working at weekends or even Bank Holidays, (for weddings etc.) but it will definitely involve late-night openings – working on into the evening at least one day per week.

TOP TIP

Saturday is a normal working day in a hairdressing salon or barber's shop. Salon work may involve late-night working or training as well.

Career opportunities in the industry

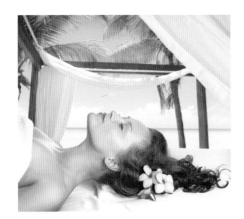

A wide range of job opportunities are available in the hairdressing and barbering industry with the obvious ones being those in hairdressing salons and barber shops. There are many other opportunities if you want to do more than just work in a salon, and even more if you want to use your qualification and travel.

- Top hotels around the world are very in-tune with the needs of their customers and are experts in providing the best in personal services. They will have lavish spas, health centres and beauty salons, catering for every need.

- Cruising is now becoming an affordable luxury for many people and all cruise liners have hair and beauty salons to cater for the needs of their passengers.

- Health farms and spas offer a wide range of jobs, mainly for beauty therapists, but there are also opportunities for hairdressers and barbers too.

- Airports around the world are busier than ever and many offer a one-stop-shop approach to the provision of services. Alongside shopping malls, coffee shops, bars, restaurants and duty-frees are barber shops and hairdressing salons.

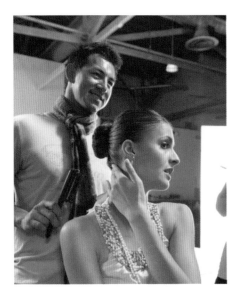

- Session stylists are another form of freelance hairdresser. There are always opportunities for the ambitious stylist in film, theatre and television.

- Session stylists are also needed in the fashion and photographic industry. These fast-moving jobs will appeal to those who want a career at the cutting-edge of fashion and innovation.

- The ever increasing need for health-related services for the elderly, retired or infirm includes hairdressing as a standard service. There are growing opportunities for hairdressers in this sector.

Other related opportunities

- Field technician/sales support for a manufacturing company – a minimum of four years as a hairdresser is needed, but this role provides a popular route for using your skills with a big name like L'Oreal, Wella or Goldwell.

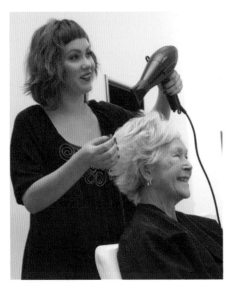

- Wholesaler, wholesale supplies – another opportunity to work on the supply side of the business, promoting and supporting sales in wholesale outlets, trade exhibitions and representative roles.

- Teaching – stylists with a minimum of five years' industry experience may want to consider an educational future. With over 400 colleges of further education and a growing number of academy and community college status schools offering vocational courses, there is always a need for people to teach hairdressing and barbering to others.

- Trichologists (hair doctors) are specialists in hair and skin dysfunctions and disorders, providing consultation, advice and treatment.

- Working for an awarding organization, e.g. City & Guilds Institute, VTCT or the industry lead body, Habia. Stylists with experience may want to consider working on the education side, in the development, maintenance and monitoring of standards or assessment systems.

Progressing onwards in your career

If you want to make the most out of your chosen career then you must find out more about the opportunities described earlier. This table shows you where to look for more information:

Job classification	Source of information
Hotels	Company Websites: Hilton Hotels, Ramada Jarvis, Marriott Hotels, Intercontinental Hotels Group, TAJ Hotels
Cruise Liners	Company Websites: Steiner Cruises
Airports	Company Websites: British Airport Authorities, BAA
Session Stylists / Freelancers	Website and Publications: The Stage
Field Technicians	Company Websites: L'Oreal Professional, Proctor and Gamble, Schwarzkopf, Unilever, Goldwell
Wholesaler Representatives	Company Websites: Sally Supplies, Ellison's, Salon Services Publications: Hairdresser's Journal, Creative Head/HeadFirst
Teaching / Assessing	Websites: Further Education Colleges TES (Times Educational Supplement), VTCT Vocational Training Charitable Trust. City and Guilds of London Institute. Publications: TES (Times Educational Supplement)
Trichologist	Websites: Institute of Trichologists
Habia	Website: Hair and Beauty Industry Authority

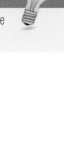

TOP TIP

The Internet is the most effective way to research jobs abroad.

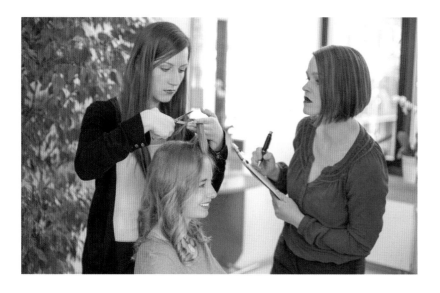

ACTIVITY

Start a training journal. Write or draw in it every day if you can: record your training and experiences, express your feelings and aspirations, draw pictures and keep it as a diary. This will become the log book of your journey towards qualifying as a hairdresser.

2 Preparing for Work

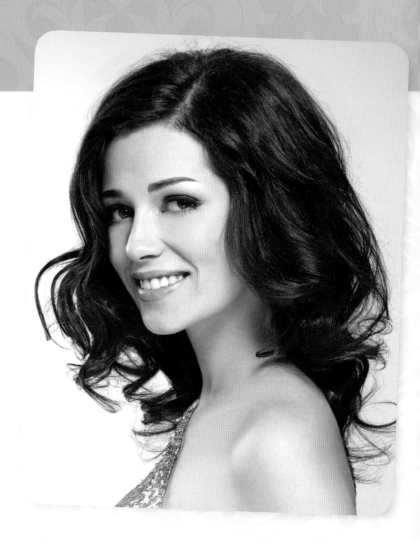

LEARNING OBJECTIVES

When you have finished this chapter you should:

◆ be able to recognize salon tools and equipment

◆ be able to prepare the salon, the tools and equipment

◆ be able to use salon tools and equipment safely

◆ know how to maintain salon tools and equipment

◆ understand the health and safety aspects relating to salon tools and equipment.

KEY TERMS

back-brushing brush

blow-dryer

ceramic straighteners

curling tongs

Data Protection Act 1998

Denman brush

detangling comb

disposable gloves

hair traps

long cutting comb

modelling blocks / mannequin heads

neck brush

paddle brush

pin-tail comb

plastic apron

portable colour processor/ accelerator

portable hood dryer

portable steamer

radial brush

sectioning clips

setting pins, grips and clips

setting rollers

short cutting comb

stock rotation

tail comb

ultraviolet radiation

UV cabinet

vented (airflow) brush

water spray

INFORMATION COVERED IN THIS CHAPTER

PRACTICAL SKILLS

Learn to use your tools for the purposes that they are intended.

Learn how to maintain your tools so that they last.

Learn how to keep them hygienically clean and safe to use.

Learn how to use items of salon equipment.

Learn how to maintain salon equipment.

Learn how to maintain the salon.

UNDERPINNING KNOWLEDGE

Know your tools and equipment and the ways that they are maintained.

Understand the ways in which you can handle them carefully and safely.

Understand the reasons why you need to keep your tools and the salon's equipment hygienically safe.

Know the salon's equipment and the ways in which it is maintained.

INTRODUCTION

If you think about a personal item that you really value, your phone, purse or wallet might spring to mind. One keeps you in touch with your friends and the other holds your money, which enables you to do things.

You will also need to include your hairdressing or barbering tools among those things that you really cherish. These items are your passport to success; they will provide you with a living for as long as you want, so make sure you look after them.

Tools and equipment

This section takes you through a typical hairdressing or barbering kit and then looks at a range of salon equipment that you need to know about.

For each piece of equipment, you will see:

◆ a picture of what it looks like

◆ what the equipment is used for

◆ how hard it is to master the techniques associated with it   Easy ———◦—→ Hard

◆ how often you will be using this during your course   Rare ———◦—→ Often

◆ the services associated with the equipment

◆ how to use this piece of equipment

◆ how the item is maintained.

Your personal tools and equipment

Long cutting comb (long, parallel body, two sets of teeth)   Used for:

◆ sectioning hair for services or conditioning treatments

◆ detangling shorter, layered hair

◆ putting partings in.

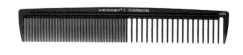

How difficult is it to use?

How often will I be using this item during my training?

Skill difficulty

Frequency of use during course

Easy ———◦—→ Hard   Rare ———◦—→ Often

This type of comb may be more difficult to handle than a shorter cutting comb as it may be quite large for a smaller hand. It is worth persevering though, as you will be using this comb a lot more when you start cutting. You will find that it is good for sectioning hair and the extra length makes it easier to hold.

Services associated with this item	Maintenance
◆ Dressing out.	✓ Remove hair and debris from teeth after use.
◆ General combing and detangling.	✓ Wash in hot, soapy water and towel dry.
◆ Combing through setting and styling products for even application.	✓ Place in Barbicide™ jar when not in use.
◆ Some conditioning treatments.	✓ Rinse and dry after Barbicide™ and before using.
◆ Sectioning for colouring.	✓ Alternatively, place in **UV cabinet** for 15 minutes then turn over for another 15 minutes.
	✗ Do not use it if it has fallen to the floor.
	✗ Do not put in your pocket – it is unhygienic and it may bend and not re-straighten.
	✗ Do not use if it has broken or missing teeth.

For detangling: A long-backed cutting comb with two sets of teeth is useful for detangling when a detangling comb is unavailable. You can comb a client's hair at the styling unit after shampooing and conditioning.

For sectioning: The main purpose for the cutting comb is the sectioning aspect during cutting and other technical services. Sectioning is usually quite hard to master, but with practice, you will find that this comb is one of the most important items in your kit.

Short cutting comb (short, parallel body, 2 sets of teeth)   Used for:

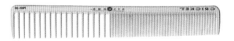

- sectioning hair for services
- detangling short hair
- putting partings in.

How difficult is it to use?   How often will I be using this item during my training?

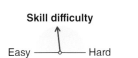

Skill difficulty

Easy ——————— Hard

Frequency of use during course

Rare ————→ Often

You will use this comb every day. This type of cutting comb is easier to use than the longer comb as it fits in the hand better. You do need to get used to using both types as they each have specific benefits. The shorter cutting comb is as strong as the longer comb although it does lack some of the larger comb's benefits. A shorter comb is *not* suitable for detangling anything more than short hair.

HEALTH & SAFETY

Combs should always be clean and ready to use; make sure that all hair and debris is removed and that they have been immersed in Barbicide for at least 30 minutes.

Services involved with this item	Maintenance
◆ Dressing out.	✓ Remove hair and debris from teeth after use.
◆ Applying styling products.	✓ Wash in hot, soapy water and towel dry.
◆ Sectioning for colouring.	✓ Place in Barbicide™ jar when not in use.
◆ Combing through temporary colours.	✓ Rinse and dry after Barbicide™ and before using.
	✓ Alternatively, place in UV cabinet for 15 minutes then turn over for another 15 minutes.
	✗ Do not use it if it has fallen to the floor.
	✗ Do not put in your pocket – it is unhygienic and may bend and not re-straighten.
	✗ Do not use if it has broken or missing teeth.

Tools and equipment (Continued...)

Pin-tail comb (a comb with a single row of teeth and a 10cm metal spine)   Used for sectioning hair when:

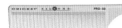

- setting and dressing out hair
- placing pin curls
- using heated styling equipment
- plaiting and twisting hair.

How difficult is it to use?   How often will I be using this item during my training?

Skill difficulty

Easy ————⊸—— Hard

Frequency of use during course

Rare ————⊸——→ Often

The pin-tail comb is quite difficult to use when you start, but it is one of the most important tools that you will own. In time, you will get used to the length of the metal pin-tail and find that you will always use it out of preference because it provides a higher degree of accuracy than other combs.

The pin-tail comb is ideal for working with small sections or meshes of hair typical in setting hair, plaiting and hair extension services. It has a narrow, parallel, steel spine that divides the hair with greater accuracy than the plastic tail comb will and this makes it far more popular for professional hairdressers. In fact, most stylists who use a pin-tail comb would never use the plastic tailed version, as it seems clumsy in comparison.

Services involved with this item	Maintenance
◆ Setting and dressing.	✓ Remove hair and debris from teeth after use.
◆ Putting hair up.	✓ Wash in hot, soapy water and towel dry.
◆ Plaiting and twisting.	✓ Place in Barbicide™ jar when not in use.
◆ Colouring.	✓ Rinse and dry after Barbicide™ and before using.
◆ Hair extensions.	✓ Alternatively, place in UV cabinet for 15 minutes then turn over for another 15 minutes.
	✗ Do not put in your pocket – it is unhygienic and the comb could pierce your clothes and skin!
	✗ Do not use if it has fallen to the floor.
	✗ Do not use it if it has broken or missing teeth.

HEALTH & SAFETY

Plastic tail combs may be safer than metal pin-tail combs, but you should never put these into your pockets as it is unhygienic and will permanently bend your comb.

For sectioning: The main purpose for the pin-tail comb is precise, accurate sectioning. The narrow tip of the comb allows you to divide the hair in any direction and its rounded edge enables you to run it across the surface of the scalp without causing the client any discomfort.

The first and second finger on one side of the comb's back and the thumb on the other hold the comb firmly. This holding position enables the stylist to turn their hand at the wrist, with palms facing downwards, which introduces the teeth of the comb to the hair, or palms upwards, which introduces the metal spine towards the hair. This comb's flexibility enables:

- ◆ horizontal sections to be taken easily

- ◆ hair to be divided into any mesh thickness

- ◆ sectioned hair to be combed to remove tangles

- ◆ a roller to be introduced to the ends of the hair and wound in during setting

- ◆ the body of tongs or straighteners to be introduced to the hair and styled

- ◆ a single weft of hair to be handled and fixed into position in plaiting, twisting and long hair work.

HEALTH & SAFETY

Pin-tail combs are very sharp and should never be put into your pocket as they will easily pierce through clothing and your skin!

Tail comb (A single row of teeth within a fixed plastic body and integrated tail)   Used for sectioning hair when:

- ◆ setting and dressing out hair

- ◆ placing pin curls

- ◆ using heated styling equipment

- ◆ plaiting and twisting hair.

How difficult is it to use?   How often will I be using this item during my training?

Skill difficulty

Easy ——————— Hard

Frequency of use during course

Rare ——————— Often

The plastic tail comb is slightly easier to handle than the metal-ended pin-tail comb. However, it is clumsier and your sectioning will not be quite as accurate. If you get used to the pin-tail comb first there will be no reason to use this comb other than as a spare when you need it.

The solid backed tail-comb is not as popular or used as often as the pin-tail comb. It is not that it is any more difficult to master than the pin-tail comb and in many respects it is more durable as the comb is made from one piece of plastic.

Hairdressers, and barbers for that matter, tend to get used to a relatively small number of *hero* items that will do a large number of jobs. This comb duplicates many of the applications that the pin-tail comb does, but it does lack the same precision and accuracy needed for sectioning, setting, long hair work, plaiting and twisting.

See pin-tail comb for information on sectioning.

Services involved with this item	Maintenance
◆ Setting and dressing.	✓ Remove hair and debris from teeth after use.
◆ Putting hair up.	✓ Wash in hot, soapy water and towel dry.
◆ Plaiting and twisting.	✓ Place in Barbicide™ jar when not in use.
◆ Hair extensions.	✓ Rinse and dry after Barbicide™ and before using.
	✓ Alternatively, place in UV cabinet for 15 minutes then turn over for another 15 minutes.
	✗ Do not put in your pocket – it is unhygienic and the comb could pierce your clothes and skin!
	✗ Do not use if it has fallen to the floor.
	✗ Do not use it if it has broken or missing teeth.

Tools and equipment (Continued...)

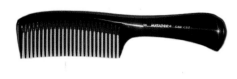

Back-brushing brush   Used for:

- applying firm support when back-brushing for dressing out

- lifting shape and maintaining balance during dressing out.

How difficult is it to use?   How often will I be using this item during my training?

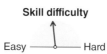
Skill difficulty

Easy ———————— Hard

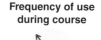
Frequency of use during course

Rare ———————— Often

Many people tend to lose their back-brushing brush at some point during their course. Look after it – it is far better to back-brush with this item rather than using a comb. You may not use it very much at Level 1, but as you progress through your training you will use it more and more!

Back-brushing is far more popular in dressing out than back-combing. It is kinder to the hair and easier to remove from the hair (by the client or the stylist) causing less *physical* damage, and is therefore the stylist's obvious choice for maintaining hair condition and quality.

The support provided by back-brushing in dressing out is virtually the same as back-combing. However, the hair is smoothed more easily, producing a neater, finished result. This brush should be considered as one of your main 'go to' *hero* tools.

TOP TIP

Plastic back-brushing brushes are really useful and you will find that you use them a lot. However, because of the closely packed bristles they tend to gather hair easily. Make sure you clean them regularly.

Services involved with this item	Maintenance
◆ Dressing out.	✓ Remove hair and debris from the bristles after use.
◆ Putting hair up.	✓ Wash in hot, soapy water and towel dry.
	✓ Place in UV cabinet for 15 minutes then turn over for another 15 minutes.
	✗ Do not put in your pocket, it is unhygienic.
	✗ Do not use if it has fallen to the floor.

Detangling comb   Used for:

- removing tangles from wet hair after shampooing and conditioning

- applying conditioning treatments evenly into longer hair.

How difficult is it to use?   How often will I be using this item during my training?

Skill difficulty

Easy ———————— Hard

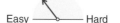
Frequency of use during course

Rare ———————→ Often

This is one of the simplest tools to use, providing you do not try to use it for precision sectioning or long hair work.

Services involved with this item	Maintenance
◆ Shampooing/conditioning.	✓ Remove hair and debris from teeth after use.
◆ Conditioning treatments.	✓ Wash in hot, soapy water and towel dry.
	✓ Place in Barbicide™ jar when not in use.
	✓ Rinse and dry after Barbicide™ and before using.
	✓ Alternatively, place in UV cabinet for 15 minutes then turn over for another 15 minutes.
	✗ Do not put this comb in your pocket – it is unhygienic.
	✗ Do not use if it has fallen to the floor.

TOP TIP

Always remember to use tools for the purpose they are intended. You will use a detangling comb every day during your training and when you have qualified.

For detangling: You can comb a client's hair after shampooing and conditioning when they have been moved back to the styling unit. Start at the ends of the hair and work upwards.

For conditioning treatments: The comb is used in the same way as detangling, but for the purpose of spreading conditioner through the hair evenly so that all porous areas are treated.

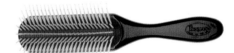

Denman brush   Used for:

- ◆ blow-drying different hair lengths into smoother styles;
- ◆ achieving small amounts of lift during blow-drying;
- ◆ brushing out dry hair and moderate detangling before shampooing;
- ◆ brushing out roller marks after setting and before dressing out.

How difficult is it to use?   How often will I be using this item during my training?

Skill difficulty

Easy ———┴——— Hard

Frequency of use during course

Rare ———○——→ Often

The Denman is a multi-purpose brush and when used for general brushing and grooming it is the easiest brush to use. However, it is the main brush for blow-drying and dressing out too, and these skills are much harder to master.

TOP TIP

The Denman is the most versatile brush that you will own. They are very durable and comfortable for the clients too. You can make them last longer by making sure that you dry the rubber head after cleaning; this will help to prevent the rubber from splitting and perishing.

Services involved with this item	Maintenance
◆ Blow-drying.	✓ Remove cushioned, rubber brush head by sliding out of handle and open flat.
◆ Dressing out.	✓ Check rubber head for splits or damage.
◆ Putting hair up.	✓ Remove rows of nylon bristles from rubber head and wash bristle rows, brush head and brush back in hot, soapy water; towel dry.
◆ Detangling and general brushing prior to many other services.	✓ Place individual items in UV cabinet for 15 minutes then turn over for another 15 minutes.
	✓ Reassemble the bristle rows into the dry cushioned head and fold back into shape.
	✓ Apply a little talc to the slotted grooves and slide back into the handle.
	✗ Do not leave the cushioned head wet as the rubber will perish too quickly.

Tools and equipment (Continued...)

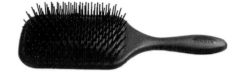

Paddle brush   Used for:

- blow-drying longer, one-length hair into smoother styles
- brushing out dry hair and moderate detangling before shampooing.

How difficult is it to use?   How often will I be using this item during my training?

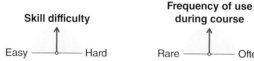

Skill difficulty

Easy ———○——— Hard

Frequency of use during course

Rare ———○——— Often

The flat paddle brush is far easier to use than a Denman. Its wide cushioned head is more stable when it is used for brushing or blow-drying. You will use a paddle brush for general brushing every day, even if you do not choose to use it for blow-drying.

The paddle brush is designed for longer hair; it has a cushioned, wide head with coarser, soft tip bristles. This makes it the most comfortable brush for detangling any length hair before shampooing and general brushing for longer hair.

If there were one brush that should be recommended for use by clients on their own hair, or for their family's use, then this is it. As a general brush, it is very easy to use and lasts a long time; as a blow-drying brush it is slightly harder to master, but the wider, flatter head helps to control the hair during drying.

TOP TIP

Paddle brushes are really suited for longer or thicker hair types. You can use a paddle brush from any angle, with any side as your leading edge, so they are highly versatile.

Services involved with this item	Maintenance
◆ Blow-drying.	✓ Remove hair and debris from teeth after use.
◆ Detangling and general brushing prior to many other services.	✓ Wash in hot, soapy water and towel dry.
	✓ Place brush in UV cabinet for 15 minutes then turn over for another 15 minutes.
	✗ Do not leave the cushioned head wet as the rubber will quickly perish.
	✗ Do not use if it has fallen to the floor.

For blow-drying: The width of the brush head requires the user to place sections of their hair onto the brush before they can dry them. In many ways this removes a lot of the problems that someone without hairdressing experience could encounter because:

- it uses both hands and stops them from using the brush to twist the hair over the bristles
- it is a wider brush with wider teeth; it is easier to hold and doesn't tangle as easily as narrower brushes
- it helps the hair to dry faster than narrower, bristled brushes.

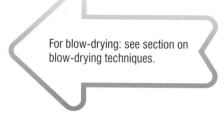

For blow-drying: see section on blow-drying techniques.

Vented (airflow) brush   Used for:

◆ blow-drying short, medium and longer length hair

◆ achieving small amounts of lift during blow-drying

◆ brushing out roller marks after setting and before dressing out.

How difficult is it to use?   How often will I be using this item during my training?

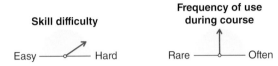

Skill difficulty

Easy ———————— Hard

Frequency of use during course

Rare ———————— Often

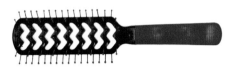

The vented brush is harder to use than a paddle or Denman brush. This is because it has narrower plastic bristles and a hollow brush back that hair can easily get caught in. However, when you have mastered the holding and drying technique, you will find that it enables wet hair to dry much faster than any other type of brush. If you get used to it early on, you will find that it is one of the most frequently used brushes and will cut down your timings for blow-drying hair.

The cheaper versions of this brush are made from one piece and have narrow, strong bristles that are 'planted' directly into its handle. The more expensive versions have a soft-touch handle, which improves the grip, so has less chance of ending up on the floor.

One of its disadvantages is that it can be painful for the client if the stylist has had little practice or training in using it, as it is very light in weight and can lead to a stylist being heavy handed in use. Vented brush bristles are quite stiff and they can scratch the client's scalp during use, especially the first row of bristles, as these engage with the head first when picking up hair. Because of this, a vented brush is not recommended for general brushing and detangling.

The vented brush does have one main advantage over all other brushes, i.e. the speed at which it can dry hair during blow-drying, which is due to the brush's design. The brush head has a skeleton construction, which allows the flow of air from a **blow-dryer** to pass through the hair rather than being deflected off the surface of the brush head. This simple scientific benefit speeds up drying by up to a half, and in a busy salon this has obvious attractions.

Services involved with this item	Maintenance
◆ Blow-drying.	✓ Remove hair and debris from teeth after use.
	✓ Wash in hot, soapy water and towel dry.
	✓ Place brush in UV cabinet for 15 minutes then turn over for another 15 minutes.
	✗ Do not use if it has fallen to the floor.

TOP TIP

Avoid using a vented brush for detangling as it can easily catch and tug on the client's hair.

HEALTH & SAFETY

Vented brushes have very stiff bristles and this can be quite painful for clients with sensitive scalps.

Tools and equipment (Continued...)

Radial brush   There are two types, and a typical radial brush set of either type will have up to five different sizes.

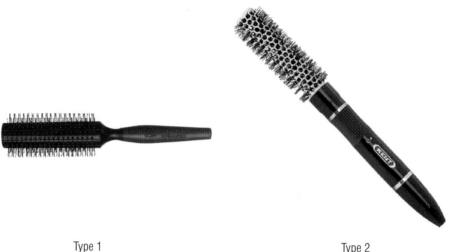

Type 1   Type 2

Used for blow-drying hair:

- ◆ on short, medium and longer length hair

- ◆ to achieve strong lift and root movement

- ◆ to create end curl and movement in any length of hair.

How difficult is it to use?   How often will I be using this item during my training?

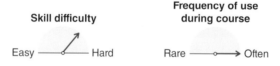

Radial brushes are the most difficult blow-drying tools to use, but they create the best blow-dried effects. You will have to master the technique for using them and there will be times when the hair catches and knots around them. You might be embarrassed but don't give up; good blow-drying skills are essential for a true professional. Use the different size brushes every day: practice makes perfect!

The radial brush is the only tool for adding volume and curl into a blow-dried style. They are very durable and designed to be continually heated and cooled by a dryer. Admittedly, there are different qualities and the brush set that you start with may need replacing within a few years, but a more expensive set will last you for most of your hairdressing career.

There are two main types of radial brush as illustrated above:

- ◆ Type 1 has strong, plastic teeth like a vented brush. This type of brush is quicker to use and dries hair more quickly than type 2. It is designed to be used in a similar way to a Denman or vent brush, in that it is held in one hand while the blow-dryer is held in the other. During use, the leading edge or rows of bristles are engaged with the hair to pick it up and roll it around the brush's body while it is dried into shape. This type of brush is good for providing lift and end curl.

◆ Type 2 has softer bristles that are positioned closer together in a 'bottle brush' design. These bristles try to prevent the hair from falling inwards, i.e. lying closer to the brush's body. Therefore, the type 2 brush works in a similar way to a setting roller, providing a much stronger root lift, volume and end curl than the type 1. However, because the hair is more easily tangled on this type of brush, you need two hands free during the blow dry so that you can pick up and position the ends around the brush carefully before drying into style.

Services involved with this item	Maintenance
◆ Blow-drying.	✓ Remove hair and debris from teeth after use.
	✓ Wash in hot, soapy water and towel dry.
	✓ Place brush in UV cabinet for 15 minutes then turn over for another 15 minutes.
	✗ Do not put in your pocket, it is unhygienic.
	✗ Do not use if it has fallen to the floor.

TOP TIP

Radial brushes are difficult to master – start learning with type 1 and the others will be easy to use.

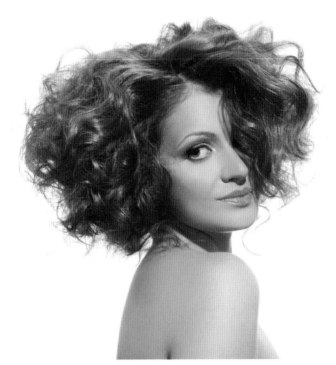

A radial brush is the best tool for adding volume and curl into a blow-dried style.

Tools and equipment (Continued...)

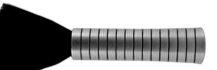

Neck brush   Used for:

◆ brushing hair clippings away from the skin after the stylist has cut the client's hair.

How difficult is it to use?   How often will I be using this item during my training?

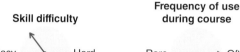

Skill difficulty   **Frequency of use during course**

Easy ——————— Hard   Rare ——————→ Often

The neck brush is the only brush suitable for removing hair clippings after the client has had their hair cut. It is easy to use as the long, soft, flexible bristles will quickly *sweep* away any debris. You will probably use this brush every day.

Unfortunately, the longer bristle neck brushes are prone to shedding hairs and becoming misshapen, particularly if they are not looked after carefully. As an alternative you can buy a shorter length bristled brush but these are not as comfortable for the client, although they will last longer.

After the stylist has finished the cut, you can use the neck brush around the neckline of the cutting collar, *before* it is removed. If the stylist has trimmed a beard or moustache you will need to gently *sweep* around the chin and cheeks too. Always remember to do this; the clients will be very uncomfortable if you do not.

TOP TIP

Your clients need to feel comfortable throughout their hairdressing or barbering service. The more times you brush away the loose clippings the happier and more comfortable they will be.

Services involved with this item	Maintenance
◆ Cutting women's hair.	✓ Wash in hot, soapy water and towel dry.
◆ Cutting men's hair.	✓ Place brush in UV cabinet for 15 minutes then turn over for another 15 minutes.
◆ Cutting beards and moustaches.	✗ Do not allow the brush to dry with bristles in a bent position; it will shorten the brush's life dramatically.
	✗ Do not use if it has fallen to the floor.

Cutting collar   Used for:

◆ protecting the client from clippings going down their neck during cutting services

◆ keeping the client comfortable during cutting services

◆ keeping clothes smooth under the cap or gown during cutting, and providing a flatter base on which to cut and improve cutting accuracy.

How difficult is it to use?   How often will I be using this item during my training?

Skill difficulty   **Frequency of use during course**

Easy ◄——————— Hard   Rare ——————→ Often

The cutting collar is an invaluable piece of equipment and any hairdresser or barber that doesn't use one is being unprofessional in their work. It provides PPE for the client and helps to maintain accuracy during the hair cut by either providing a base to establish balance and do freehand cutting against, or by keeping clothes out of the way, which enables the stylist to see the position of the shoulders in relation to the cut length of the hairstyle.

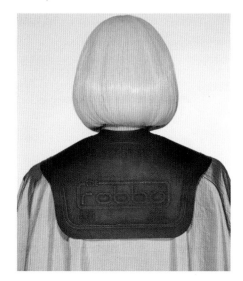

Cutting collars vary dramatically in price and quality. A typical college kit item will be at the entry level quality and may not last the length of the course. The more expensive versions are made from materials that are more durable and have weighted fronts that help to keep cumbersome clothes flat. These will last for several years providing they are properly maintained.

Services involved with this item	Maintenance
◆ Cutting women's hair.	✓ Wash in hot, soapy water and towel dry.
◆ Cutting men's hair.	✗ Do not put in direct sunlight or place on anything hot, as this will change the material's properties, causing it to distort or split.
◆ Cutting beards and moustaches.	

Tools and equipment (Continued...)

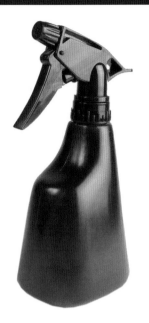

Water spray   Used for keeping hair damp during:

◆ setting and putting rollers in

◆ blow-drying techniques.

How difficult is it to use?   How often will I be using this item during my training?

Skill difficulty	Frequency of use during course
Easy ◄——o—— Hard	Rare ——o——► Often

Apply a light misting to the hair during:

◆ rollering – so that the hair being set doesn't have the chance to form an un-stretched 'beta keratin' state before going under a dryer

◆ blow-drying – this stops the hair from drying out and will make the blow dry last longer.

Services involved with this item	Maintenance
◆ Cutting.	◆ Remove spray top and wash bottle and spray in hot soapy water; rinse with clean water and dry with a towel.
◆ Setting.	◆ Rinse out stale water often and replace with fresh, clean water.
◆ Perming.	

TOP TIP

Check that the nozzle is working properly and adjust so that it does not soak the hair. Lightly mist the hair as and when required.

Sectioning clips   We use two types – crocodile clips and flat clips.

Used for sectioning and fixing hair during:

◆ blow-drying

◆ setting and dressing

◆ long hair work

◆ plaiting and twisting

◆ colouring.

How difficult is it to use?   How often will I be using this item during my training?

Skill difficulty	Frequency of use during course
Easy ◄——o—— Hard	Rare ——o——► Often

TOP TIP

Keep your water spray filled with fresh water. Stale water can smell and can even make the client's hair feel greasier.

There are two types of sectioning clips and each does a different job. Both types are relatively easy to use and each has advantages and disadvantages.

The crocodile clip is good for holding lots of heavy hair, i.e. bulk and weight.

Advantages:

◆ has powerful jaws that are great for holding large amounts of hair or dense, heavy hair out of the way

◆ good for holding longer hair up and out of the way.

Disadvantages:

◆ the clip is quite vicious and can easily be placed too tightly and will then pull or catch on the client's hair

◆ doesn't last as long as a flat clip; the springs tend to give out quicker so has to be thrown away.

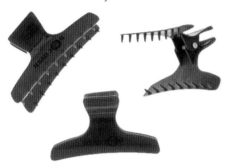

Crocodile clips

> **TOP TIP**
>
> Different types of clips do different jobs. You need to have both – the crocodile clips for large amounts of thick or heavy hair and the flat clips for precision sectioning and hair placement.

The flat clip is good for delicate or precision placement and better organization of work.

Advantages:

◆ useful on shorter or layered hair

◆ easier to remove and doesn't catch on the client's hair; far more comfortable to wear

◆ clips the hair parallel to the head so it is easier to judge balance during cutting

◆ does not crush or distort dry, styled hair, therefore better for hair-ups, plaiting, twisting and tonging or straightening hair.

Disadvantages:

◆ not as strong as the crocodile clip so will not hold heavy hair securely

◆ more prone to breaking.

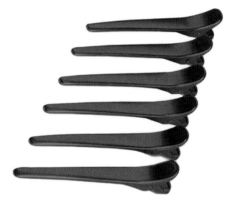

Flat clips

Services involved with this item	Maintenance
◆ Setting and dressing.	✓ Wash in hot, soapy water and towel dry.
◆ Plaiting and twisting.	✓ Place brush in UV cabinet for 15 minutes then turn over for another 15 minutes.
◆ Putting hair up.	✗ Do not use if it has fallen to the floor.
◆ Conditioning treatments.	
◆ Consultations during examination.	
◆ Colouring.	

> **TOP TIP**
>
> Only use a crocodile clip on heavy, dense or thicker, longer hair. Never use on finer, more delicate hair types.

Tools and equipment (Continued...)

Colouring set (brush, bowl and measuring flask)   Used for:

◆ control and accuracy in colouring or lightening small or narrower root areas

◆ woven highlights

◆ partial colouring techniques.

How difficult is it to use?   How often will I be using this item during my training?

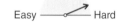

Skill difficulty

Frequency of use during course

Easy ——————— Hard   Rare ——————→ Often

The standard college kit colouring set is very durable and will last you for years. This classic brush set is still the best, although newer versions may look more appealing with colourful, larger bowls, wider brush tips and chamfered edges. If you have the choice, choose a brush that is conventionally narrow like the one shown on the left. These brushes last longer and are less prone to misshaping or bending. Choose a bowl that has a rubberized (neoprene) grip to stop it sliding about on your work trolley when you try to use it.

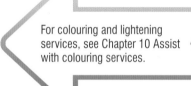

For colouring and lightening services, see Chapter 10 Assist with colouring services.

Services involved with this item	Maintenance
◆ Colouring.	✓ Wash items in hot, soapy water and towel dry.
◆ Bleaching.	✓ Never leave colour on the brush around the top of the bristles; it will affect the next colour that you use with it.
◆ Highlighting.	✗ Never leave developer in the measuring flask.

Disposable gloves (nitrile or vinyl)   Standard PPE within the salon and must be worn in all situations where hands may come into contact with chemicals; prevents the risk of dermatitis. Used for:

◆ shampooing

◆ conditioning

◆ applying colour

◆ mixing and handling any chemicals.

How difficult is it to use?   How often will I be using this item during my training?

Skill difficulty

Frequency of use during course

Easy ◄——————— Hard   Rare ——————→ Often

TOP TIP

Clean colouring brushes thoroughly, making sure that you get to the base of the bristles and remove any previously used product.

There are two forms of safe disposable gloves. The nitrile (blue) glove is closer fitting and provides better sensitivity when doing intricate work. However, the nitrile glove has a grip more like rubber so it can grab the client's hair during shampooing and conditioning. The vinyl glove has more slip, so is far better for shampooing and conditioning but less useful in technical services like colouring. Both are easy to use and you would be advised to wear both types depending on the work you are doing.

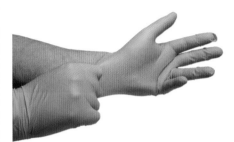

Services involved with this item	Maintenance
◆ Shampooing and conditioning.	None – a new pair is worn for each service/treatment.
◆ Conditioning treatments.	
◆ Colouring – mixing and application.	
◆ Lightening – mixing and application.	
◆ Perming – application of lotion.	
◆ Neutralizing.	

Plastic apron
Standard PPE within the salon and must be worn for all chemical treatments or services. Used for:

- applying colour

- mixing and handling any chemicals.

How difficult is it to use?   How often will I be using this item during my training?

Skill difficulty

Easy ◄———○——— Hard

Frequency of use during course

Rare ———○——► Often

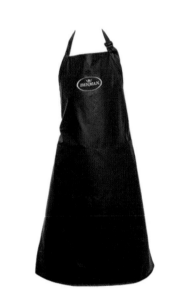

Aprons are usually made of plastic, which makes them easy to clean and light to wear. A typical hairdressing apron has adjustable neck straps to suit different heights and for extra comfort. They usually have two large front storage pockets for holding a range of hairdressing tools, gloves and accessories. Your salon will provide you with an apron.

Services involved with this item	Maintenance
◆ Conditioning treatments.	✓ Simply wipe over with a cloth to remove light staining.
◆ Colouring.	✓ Wash in hot soapy water to remove heavier soiling; blot dry with a towel and hang up so that creases fall out.
◆ Lightening.	✗ Do not put in the washing machine/tumble dryer as it will crease the garment.
◆ Perming.	
◆ Neutralizing.	

TOP TIP

- Wear disposable non-latex gloves when rinsing, shampooing, colouring, bleaching, etc.

- Dry your hands thoroughly with a soft cotton or paper towel.

- Moisturize after washing your hands, as well as at the start and end of each day. It's easy to miss fingertips, finger webs and wrists.

- Change gloves between clients. Make sure you don't contaminate your hands when you take them off.

- Check your skin regularly for early signs of dermatitis.

Salon equipment

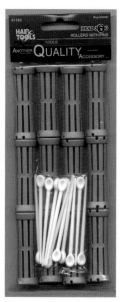

Setting rollers or curlers

For setting, see Chapter 8
Dressing, plaiting and
twisting hair.

Setting rollers   Setting rollers come in many sizes and are used for:

- setting hair – providing lift or volume, movement or curl
- wet setting rollers
- dry setting /heated rollers.

How difficult is it to use?   How often will I be using this item during my training?

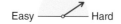

Skill difficulty

Easy ———— Hard

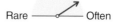

**Frequency of use
during course**

Rare ———— Often

Most learners find the technique of setting quite difficult and there is a good reason for that. With most skills you get better as you get to a higher level. Unfortunately, with rollering it is either right or wrong, at any level. Most learners find heated rollers easier to use and comb out than wet setting rollers, therefore heated rollers get used more often.

The skills relating to setting and dressing out are related to other aspects such as blow-drying and the use of heated styling equipment. Setting hair, i.e. rollering, is quite difficult for any new student hairdresser to master. A lot of your training will be spent applying rollers to a mannequin head/practice block. The technique is covered in depth in Chapter 8, however, the three hardest things to master are:

- getting the points of the hair around the roller without buckling the ends (fish-hooks)
- understanding the correct size of roller to use to create the effect that you want on a variety of hair textures
- dressing out the hair after the rollers have been removed.

Services involved with this item	Maintenance
◆ Setting (wet and dry hair).	✓ Remove traces of styling product or hair by brushing over the surface of the roller.
◆ Hair ups.	✓ Wash all rollers in hot, soapy water and towel dry.
◆ Finishing off a long hair blow-dry with heated rollers.	✗ Do not use heated rollers without checking the lead and plug beforehand.
	✗ Do not use heated rollers wound down to a client's scalp without cotton wool in between (you may burn the client).

TOP TIP

Setting lotions and other styling products become dried onto the rollers each time they are used. This builds up a dirty layer making the rollers unhygienic to use. They will need regular washing and drying before use.

Setting pins, grips and clips Used for:

◆ Pins – securing rollers into wet hair while setting

◆ Grips – securing dry hair into position for all sorts of hairdressings and hair-ups, e.g. pleats, plaits, knots, rolls, twists, folds, etc.

◆ Clips – pin curling – a setting technique where clips often form part of the overall set hairstyle.

How difficult is it to use?　　How often will I be using this item during my training?

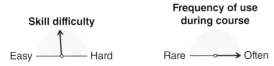

Skill difficulty

Easy ———————— Hard

Frequency of use during course

Rare ———————→ Often

Setting pins are easy to use. It's the grips and clips or the techniques associated with them that are difficult to master. You will be using at least one of these items on a daily basis.

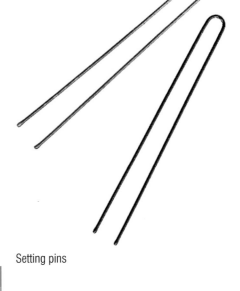

Setting pins

Services involved with this item	Maintenance
◆ Setting (pins and clips).	✓ The metal pins, grips and clips have no method for cleaning and maintaining hygiene.
◆ Plaiting and twisting (grips and clips).	✓ Plastic pins are often used in salons instead of metal pins, and these can be washed in hot soapy water and dried with a towel before putting away .
◆ Long hair-ups (grips).	

For setting, see Chapter 8 Dressing, plaiting and twisting hair.

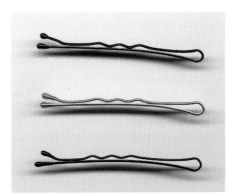

Grips

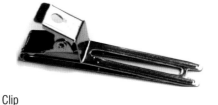

Clip

TOP TIP

Pins, clips and grips are small fiddly items that can drop on the floor, particularly when you try to handle them. Never use a clip, pin or grip if it has been on the floor; if it cannot be cleaned it must be binned.

Salon equipment (Continued...)

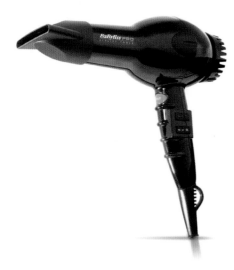

Blow-dryer and diffuser attachment
Used for blow-drying hair with a nozzle to produce:

◆ smoother effects

◆ volume

◆ styles with curl or movement.

Used with the diffuser attachment for:

◆ finger drying

◆ scrunch drying (wavy or curly hair).

How difficult is it to use?	How often will I be using this item during my training?
Skill difficulty	**Frequency of use during course**

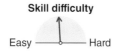

Easy —————— Hard   Rare ————→ Often

A blow-dryer is quite difficult to master across all the styling techniques. Admittedly, some techniques are a lot easier than others, and most learners can pick up the flat brush techniques and finger drying quite quickly. However, being able to blow-dry with radial brushes and get the set-like results takes a lot of practice.

The blow-dryer is one of the most commonly used items of equipment in the salon. There is a huge range of models available with a variety of power outputs, speeds and heat settings. The latest ionic dryers can even reduce the flyaway effect that is produced by static electricity when hair is heated in a colder environment.

A good professional hair blow-dryer should:

◆ have at least two speeds and two heat settings

◆ have different shaped nozzles to channel the heat onto the brush or comb

◆ have a lead long enough for it not to tangle around the chair or client

◆ be powerful enough to dry damp hair quickly (1300–1500w)

◆ have a 'cool shot' button to enable hot hair to be fixed (set) into shape around a brush

◆ not be too long so that it is balanced in the hand and can be held away from the client's hair during drying

◆ be light enough so that it can be manipulated easily and used for long periods without fatigue

◆ be quiet enough so that it allows natural conversation with the client.

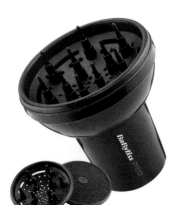

For blow-drying or finger drying, see Chapter 7 Styling and finishing hair.

Services involved with this item	Maintenance
◆ Blow-drying.	✓ Blow-dryers of all qualities are made from tough durable plastics. They need little maintenance although you do need to take care when wrapping the lead around the dryer.
◆ Finger drying.	✗ Never wash or make the dryer wet; simply wipe over the casing and leads with a dry cloth.

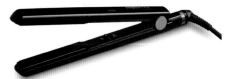

Ceramic straighteners   Used for:

◆ smoothing and straightening hair after blow-drying

◆ forming waves, volume or curls on dry hair.

How difficult is it to use?   How often will I be using this item during my training?

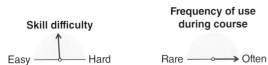

Skill difficulty

Easy ——————— Hard

Frequency of use during course

Rare ———→ Often

Most people get the hang of using straighteners for smoothing hair very quickly. Straighteners can get very hot, so always start with a lower heat setting and use heat protection to prevent damage to the client's hair. Learning to use them for waving and curling does take a lot longer to master but you could always use tongs for this purpose anyway.

Services involved with this item	Maintenance
◆ Blow-drying.	✓ Heated styling tools are made to be tough, so like blow-dryers they too are very durable.
◆ Putting hair up.	✓ They need little maintenance, although you do need to take care when wrapping the lead around the body of the straighteners. Remember to leave plenty of slack in the cable, otherwise tight coiling will shorten their life considerably.
◆ Smoothing, styling and curling hair.	✓ Make sure that any build-up of styling products on the surface of the hot plates is removed with a scouring pad before they are plugged in and used.
	✓ Use a heat mat or purpose-built holder when they are hot or in use. Leave them to cool down fully before putting away.
	✗ Do not coil the flex around the ceramic plates, this will work the flex loose and is extremely dangerous.
	✗ Do not wash them or make them wet; simply wipe over the plastic handle and leads with a dry cloth.

Salon equipment (Continued...)

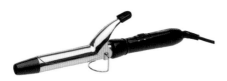

Curling tongs   Used for:

- forming wave, volume or curls on dry hair.

How difficult is it to use?   How often will I be using this item during my training?

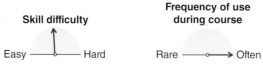

Curling tongs are easier to use than straighteners. They come in different sizes for a range of curling effects. Again, similar to straighteners, they need to be used with heat protection so that they do not damage the client's hair. You may be using them on a daily basis.

Services involved with this item	Maintenance
◆ Blow-drying.	Heated styling tools need little maintenance – follow the instructions for ceramic straighteners on page 37.
◆ Putting hair up.	
◆ Dressing out hair.	

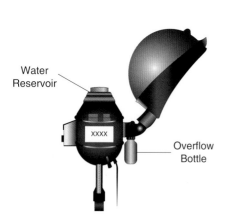

Water Reservoir

Overflow Bottle

Portable steamer   Used for:

- speeding up lightening processes involving lightener

- speeding up and helping conditioning treatments to penetrate the hair.

How difficult is it to use?   How often will I be using this item during my training?

Easy ———— Hard   Rare ———— Often

You need to be able to use a steamer safely – there are a number of safety issues that you need to know before you start. A steamer produces moist heat (i.e. steam) to process treatments and lightening services. The steam is very hot and will burn the client unless you adjust the heat setting when it achieves its operating temperature. Moist heat is used in bleaching processes so that the mixture is kept moist, stopping it from drying out and processing.

If the salon does a lot of lightening/bleaching services and conditioning treatments, then you will find that the steamer will be used on a daily basis.

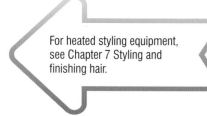

For heated styling equipment, see Chapter 7 Styling and finishing hair.

To use a steamer safely and correctly there are a number of things that you need to do:

1. Check that the steamer has been cleaned properly and that there are no traces of dried out bleach around the rim of the hood.

2. Check the water reservoir. If the water is not above the minimum level, remove the reservoir and top up with cold/cool water and replace.

3. Check the water overflow bottle and that the pipe leading to it is not blocked. If the bottle has any water left in it from the previous use, empty it down the sink and replace in the machine.

4. Check the leads and plug. If OK, switch it on and close the vents at the front. Select the pre-heat or high setting and turn the timer switch on for approximately ten minutes (the steamer needs to be ready at the point where the conditioning or lightening service is ready to be developed).

5. When the steamer has started to produce steam from beneath the plastic hood, turn the heat setting to normal or low. It will continue to produce steam but not so vigorously.

The steamer is now ready for the client's service or treatment.

6. Adjust the height of the hood so that it covers the back and the side of the client's head.

7. Readjust the time setting in accordance with the stylist's instructions.

8. Go back to check that the client is comfortable, that the overflow is working OK, and that it is not too hot. If it is hot, open the vents to allow more steam to escape.

9. Recheck with the client after 3–4 minutes to make sure they are OK.

TOP TIP

Keep the surfaces of the hot plates clean and free from product build-up, as they will grab and burn the hair next time you want to use them.

Services involved with this item	Maintenance
◆ Highlights.	✓ Make sure that the inside of the hood is cleaned before and after each use.
◆ Re-touch lightener/bleach.	✓ Check the leads and plug before use.
◆ Full headlightener/bleach.	✓ Check the water reservoir and top up if necessary.
◆ Some conditioning treatments.	✓ Turn the machine on before you need it to warm up.
	✓ Adjust the vents or the heat setting when it is boiling and producing steam.
	✓ Check the temperature when the client is sat beneath it.
	✓ Check the overflow to make sure it is not full and safe to use.
	✗ Do not allow the water level to drop below the recommended minimum limit.
	✗ Do not leave the client unattended whilst it is on.
	✗ Do not leave on a high heat setting when it is being used for a service or treatment.

HEALTH & SAFETY

Never try to clean hot surfaces; wait until they have cooled down.

TOP TIP

Always use a heat mat when you use straighteners or tongs; it will stop them from damaging the work surfaces and laminated finishes.

Salon equipment (Continued...)

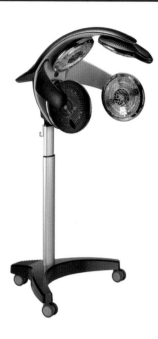

Portable hood dryer   Used for:

◆ drying a roller set.

How difficult is it to use?   How often will I be using this item during my training?

Easy ———————— Hard   Rare ——————→ Often

A hood dryer is fairly simple to use but you do need to do some safety checks before using it.

1. Check that the dryer has been cleaned properly inside and outside of the hood.

2. Check the leads and plug. If OK switch it on.

3. Turn the heat setting selector to medium.

4. Now pre-heat the dryer by turning the timer to ten minutes – the dryer should now be working.

5. Close the face visor (if fitted) and leave to heat up.

6. When the client is ready, check with the stylist to see what heat level (low-med-high) is required and adjust the heat and timer accordingly.

7. Sit the client underneath the dryer and recheck that they are comfortable and that the dryer is not too hot after a few minutes.

Services involved with this item	Maintenance
◆ Setting hair.	✓ Make sure that the inside of the hood is cleaned before and after each use.
◆ Sometimes used for colouring processes when an accelerator is not available.	✓ Check the leads and plug before use.
	✓ Turn the machine on before you need it to warm up.
	✓ Check the temperature when the client is sat beneath it.
	✗ Do not leave the client unattended whilst it is on.
	✗ Do not leave on a high heat setting when a client is sat beneath it.

Portable colour processor/accelerator   Used for:

- ◆ speeding up colouring processes;
- ◆ speeding up some conditioning treatments.

How difficult is it to use?   How often will I be using this item during my training?

Easy ——————— Hard   Rare ————→ Often

An accelerator produces dry heat to process treatments and colouring services. The machine will get very hot if the settings are not monitored closely during a colour's development. As this is another electrical piece of equipment, you will need to perform the same checks before it is used as with previous equipment.

If the salon does a lot of colouring and conditioning treatments, then you will find that the colour accelerator will be used on a daily basis. To use a colour accelerator safely and correctly, follow the steps below:

1. Check that the heat radiant panels/arms have been cleaned properly; both inside and outside.

2. Check the leads and plug. If OK switch it on.

3. Turn the heat setting selector to medium.

4. Now preheat the radiants by turning the timer to ten minutes – the accelerator should now be working.

5. When the client is ready, check with the stylist to see what heat level (low-med-high) is required and adjust the heat and timer accordingly.

6. Sit the client underneath the accelerator. Recheck that they are comfortable and that the dryer is not too hot after a few minutes.

Services involved with this item	Maintenance
◆ Highlights/lowlights.	✓ Make sure that the inside of the radiant panels/arms are cleaned before and after each use.
◆ Re-touch colouring.	✓ Check the leads and plug before use.
◆ Full head colouring.	✓ Turn the machine on before you need it to warm up.
◆ Some conditioning treatments.	✓ Check the temperature when the client is sitting underneath it.
	✗ Do not leave the client unattended while it is on.
	✗ Do not leave on high heat setting when it is being used for a service or treatment.

Salon equipment (Continued...)

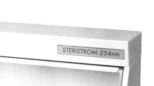

UV cabinet   Used for sterilizing tools and equipment, making them hygienically safe before they are used, e.g. scissors, razors, brushes, combs.

How difficult is it to use?   How often will I be using this item during my training?

Easy ——————— Hard   Rare ——————→ Often

A UV cabinet is the quickest way of preparing tools and equipment to make them safe and hygienic. When the cabinet is in operation, **ultraviolet radiation** is emitted from the top of the cabinet on to the items laid out on a grilled shelf below. Items are left for ten minutes and then turned over, so that the UV rays can sterilize the other side for another ten minutes.

Sterilization is the only way of killing 100 per cent of harmful bacteria. The UV cabinet will be used several times throughout the day.

To use a UV cabinet safely and correctly, follow the steps below:

1. Check that the cabinet has been cleaned properly inside and outside with antiseptic/disinfecting spray and a clean cloth.

2. Check the leads and plug.

3. Place a number of items on to the grill inside the UV cabinet.

4. Close the door and press/switch on – the timer should show and start counting down automatically.

5. When the timer goes off, open the door and turn over the items so that they can be sterilized on the other side.

6. Switch back on for a further ten minutes.

7. When the timer goes off for a second time the items are ready for use.

Services involved with this item	Maintenance
◆ Hygienic preparation of certain tools for all hairdressing and barbering services.	✓ Wipe over the grilled shelf and both inside and outside of the cabinet with an antiseptic spray and cloth before use.
	✓ Check the leads and plug regularly for deterioration or loose cables.
	✗ Do not put too many items into the cabinet at one time; make sure that they lie directly on the grill.

Modelling blocks and mannequin heads

Your training mannequin head is usually referred to as a modelling block. You will find that during your course, or certainly the early part of it, you will be using the practice block every day. The skills that you learn in the hours spent in training will not be wasted because each time that you use it you are one step closer to working on real clients.

The practice block is durable but in order for you to get the best out of it, there are some dos and don'ts. First you need to remember that they come in a range of different qualities and types. The standard ones from a wholesaler will not take a lot of harsh treatment.

Type of block	Information	Dos and don'ts
Standard modelling block.	This is the general modelling head that you will find in any wholesaler. 100 per cent human hair 30–35cm long Medium density: 230–260 hairs per square cm The hair is chemically treated and pre-coloured to mid brown. The hair is implanted backwards around the front hairline to enable the hair to be brushed or styled back away from the facial area, smoothly and without a definite parting.	✓ Cutting. ✓ Heat styling. ✓ Setting. ✓ Dressing/plaiting/twisting. ✓ Hair-ups. ✓ Colouring. ✓ Highlighting. ✓ Lightening. ✓ Perming (water wind only). ✗ Perming. ✗ Chemical relaxers.
High quality modelling block.	If you want to purchase a high-quality block, look online for the best prices. 100 per cent human hair 30–35cm long Medium density: 230–260 hairs per square cm This higher quality training head has a neck and shoulders. This makes it suitable for display work, precision cutting, styling and hair-ups; generally associated with competition work.	✓ Cutting. ✓ Heat styling. ✓ Setting. ✓ Dressing/plaiting/twisting. ✓ Hair-ups. ✓ Colouring. ✓ Highlighting. ✓ Bleaching. ✓ Perming. ✗ Chemical relaxers.
High quality male modelling block.	100 per cent human hair – large head circumference of 59cm Forward fringe implant – 20cm long High density: 260–290 hairs per square cm The head circumference is larger than the standard modelling block so there is a lot more coverage of hair over the head form, which provides a greater density and allows you to produce fringes and forward lying hairstyles. This type of block will also tolerate close clipper grades without exposing scalp/nape thin areas.	✓ Cutting. ✓ Heat styling. ✓ Setting. ✓ Dressing/plaiting/twisting. ✓ Hair-ups. ✓ Colouring. ✓ Highlighting. ✓ Bleaching. ✓ Perming. ✗ Chemical relaxers.

Salon equipment (Continued...)

Modelling blocks and mannequin heads (continued)

Type of block	Information	Dos and don'ts
Standard quality long hair modelling block	100 per cent natural hair (not necessarily human) Medium density: 230–260 hairs per square cm – 60cms long This type of block requires a lot of maintenance and will deteriorate quickly if the hair is not taken down and brushed out after each styling	✓ Hair-ups. ✓ Dressing/plaiting/twisting. ✓ Cutting. ✗ Heat styling. ✗ Setting. ✗ Colouring. ✗ Highlighting. ✗ Lightening. ✗ Perming. ✗ Chemical relaxers.
Standard clamp	All modelling blocks have a nylon/plastic clamp in the box. These types of clamps will enable you to affix the block to a table top or styling shelf.	✓ Make sure that you protect the surface of the shelf from scratches or dents by covering it with a towel or cloth first. ✗ Do not over-tighten the clamp as the screw thread area will snap off!

Modelling block care and maintenance
If you want to get the most out of your block you must look after it. Even though most blocks are made from human hair, it does not make them very durable. Heat styling with very hot straighteners will shorten its life and the handling properties of the block.

The main problems with handling are more to do with the way that the blocks are initially prepared and processed. When the block manufacturers buy hair, it has to be cleaned, coloured and stabilized. Generally, the bulk hair bought for making blocks is of Asian origin and this hair is usually black. The first part of the processing is cleaning, so in the interests of hygiene, the bulk hair is washed and sterilized and this kills off any infestations or contamination. These are strong alkaline chemicals and this tends to swell the hair, making it coarser in texture.

TOP TIP

For more specialist information, visit this supplier to the industry: www.banburypostiche.co.uk

The hair is then dyed or in some cases bleached, to produce mid browns, golden blondes or black colour options. Nevertheless, the most popular colour is brown. Finally, the hair is conditioned and pH balanced so that the cuticle flattens, which helps with brushing and combing.

All this chemical treatment makes the hair very porous and sensitive to further processing. Blocks cope better with some processes than others and as a rule of thumb they cope better with colouring and lightening than with perming or relaxing.

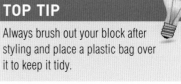

TOP TIP

Always brush out your block after styling and place a plastic bag over it to keep it tidy.

Block care and maintenance

Process, service or treatment	What you should do and why
Shampooing	◆ Always use a mild or moisturizing shampoo with cold water. This will help to stop the cuticle from becoming raised, which locks the hair together making it almost impossible to detangle.
	◆ Try to get someone to hold the block in the basin so that you can run the water down through the lengths.
	◆ Avoid using rotary massage technique; this will make the hair matted again, making it difficult to detangle. Use effleurage or squeeze between your palms instead.
Conditioning	◆ Always use an anti-oxidant or frequent use conditioner. This will fill damaged sites along the hair shaft and fill areas of torn or missing cuticle, helping you to detangle afterwards.
Detangling	◆ Always use a wide tooth comb; never use a pin-tail or narrow toothed cutting combs.
	◆ Always start at the lower nape area first, nearer the points of the hair, and remove these tangles first. Then work slowly back towards the mid lengths and root area last. The hair is going to be difficult to comb even if it hasn't been coloured or lightened, so you need to make the job easier for yourself.
Blow-drying	◆ Always dry the block off well beforehand. Squeeze excess moisture into a towel without using a rubbing action as this will make the hair matted and lock the hair together.
	◆ Avoid overheating the hair when using flat, paddle or radial brushes as this will raise the cuticle and damage the hair further. This will create problems for the next time you shampoo the block as the hair shaft will be swollen and the cuticle raised.
Heated styling equipment	◆ Always prep the hair first by using a heat protection. This will extend the life of your block by helping to maintain it in a reasonable condition.
Dressing out (after setting)	◆ Setting the block in rollers doesn't create any problems but avoid back-combing during the dressing out stage. Back-combing is potentially more damaging on any type of hair than back-brushing, so you are likely to create longer term problems and shorten the life of your block.
Plaiting – twists, cornrows, braids	◆ Always remove the plaits after your training session; never leave them in overnight. When small plaits are left in for any length of time they tend to damage or distort/kink the hair and this will limit your styling options in the future.
Colouring and lightening	◆ Practice heads will tolerate most colouring and lightening techniques although they do not respond well to higher strength developers. Lightening the hair to extra light blond won't work – the hair will break off long before it reaches your target shade.
Styling products	◆ Avoid using any firm-hold styling products on your block such as gels, hairsprays, waxes and pomades. Blocks tend to have porous hair and this can make them difficult to manage after styling products have been applied.

Setting up tools and equipment at the start of the day

As a professional, you must make sure that you are ready to provide the services to the clients at their appointed time. You cannot wait for people to turn up then think about what you need to do – you have to make sure that you have anticipated what will be needed and have made the necessary preparations for the following:

◆ perming rods, end papers, tensioning strips, setting rollers, neck wool and barrier cream are ready in the trolley trays

◆ brushes and combs are sterilized and ready for use

◆ colouring materials, bowls, brushes, foils or meshes are available

◆ gowns and towels are washed, clean and fresh

◆ hand dryers and heated equipment are ready for use at the styling units.

Everything has to run to time in the salon or barber's shop; the stylists or barbers need to think about what they are going to do and you need to think about the things they might need. Most things are prepared in advance. For example, gowns and towels are in continual use. Salons and barbers' shops usually have more than they would use in one day so that they can make laundry processes cost effective. On the other hand, a salon or shop would not normally have heated tongs or straighteners for every senior member of staff. This is due in part to the likelihood that not everyone will need the same pieces of equipment at the same time, and partly because many stylists may use their own items of equipment. In either event, it does not matter to whom the equipment belongs; if it is used within the salon it has to be made ready and safe for use.

TOP TIP

There are always things to do in the salon if you are not busy. Why not get the perming rods out and check the rubbers to see if any have perished? Replace damaged, weakened or overstretched rubbers with new ones. You could take the curlers and rods out of the trolley trays and give them a good clean. While you are doing this, do not forget to clean the trays as well!

ACTIVITY

Your salon will have its own procedures for getting things ready. Check with your supervisor how you should prepare these items then complete the activity by copying the table below and adding the missing information.

Salon materials	Where are they kept?	How are they cleaned and prepared?	How long will they take to prepare?
setting rollers			
perming rods			
tensioning strips			
brushes			
combs			
colouring bowls and brushes			
gowns, towels and cutting collars			

You can see from the activity that these preparations take time. It would be unprofessional to wait for the client to arrive before doing them. Now, for each of the listed items answer the following questions.

1. What would happen if these preparations were not carried out beforehand?
2. What could happen if they were not done at all?

Trolleys and trays

The first job of the day is sorting out and preparing the trolley trays and because they are in continual use their contents may need to be changed several times a day.

◆ Perming curlers are colour-coded in size order and it is easier for the stylist to ask for a tray to be made up of red/blue and blue/grey curlers than some large ones and some smaller. Nevertheless, before they can be used they must be thoroughly washed and scrubbed in hot soapy water to remove all traces of perming chemicals. After washing, they need to be dried thoroughly and any broken or weak rubbers should be replaced.

◆ Setting rollers and fabric self-cling rollers are also colour-coded in size order. These can also be washed, scrubbed and dried in a similar way to perming curlers and placed in a UV cabinet.

◆ Colouring materials such as bowls and brushes need to be washed and scrubbed. They can be placed in a UV cabinet when they have been dried. The stylist will tell you the different lengths of foils or meshes that they need.

◆ Salon pins, grips, etc. are easily spilled and it is very wasteful to throw them away, but if they have been on the floor they cannot be used because of the risk of cross-infection.

However, just cleaning the trolleys in the morning is not enough. Salon trolleys are used as multipurpose workstations throughout the day and the stylists will be using them when setting hair, blow-drying, colouring and perming. With all this use, trolleys tend to need cleaning and tidying several times during the day. Fortunately they are designed with easy cleaning in mind, and a simple disinfecting spray cleaner and cleaning cloth will do the job.

HEALTH & SAFETY

Take all possible precautions to avoid dermatitis – use protective disposable gloves whenever possible.

See Chapter 3, for more information on avoiding dermatitis.

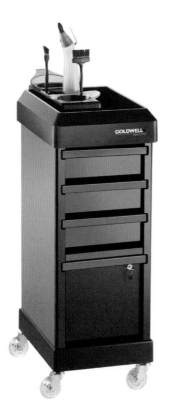

It is your job to clean and prepare the trolleys throughout the day

Get the client's records ready

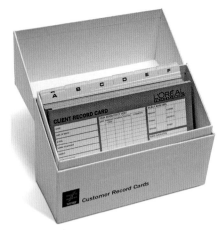

Do not let clients see each other's record cards

A salon or barber's shop keeps records of the services and treatments that the stylists provide to their clients. The records provide a way of maintaining details of treatments, tests and services, and this provides useful information for future visits. These records may be kept on record cards or electronically on a computer.

The client's records are confidential and should always be handled with care. It is very easy for this information to be left around and fall into the wrong hands. For example, imagine if a client was overheard saying that all their family was just about to go on holiday for two weeks and their details were left out in the salon. Anyone could see this information and use it maliciously!

Finding treatment records

In the past, salons created simple client records for keeping service history and contact details. Traditionally these were kept in card-index filing systems, but with the growing need to keep more information at hand many salons now use a computer. This is far more useful than the traditional card-index system because computers can find information very quickly. The way in which they search for data enables:

- ◆ easy updating and changing of information
- ◆ more information to be collected and held on file
- ◆ patterns of sales and treatments to be managed efficiently
- ◆ secure, discreet ways of keeping personal data.

See page 214 for more information on the Data Protection Act 1998.

The information kept by salons on computer is confidential and must be handled appropriately. The **Data Protection Act 1998** protects the clients from unlawful mishandling or breaches of security by the person accessing the information. Keeping client records up to date is essential because out-of-date information is useless. When you get the records for your stylist's client, remember to check the details such as address, telephone and mobile numbers with the client, so that the barber's or salon's records can be kept up to date, and that you find the right record – many people can share the same last name.

Daily salon maintenance

General salon waste The everyday items of salon waste, such as hair clippings, used colouring products, neck wool, disposable capes, etc. should be placed in an enclosed swing-lid waste bin fitted with a suitably resistant polyethylene bin liner. When the bin is full, the liner can be removed from the bin and sealed using a wire tie. Place the sealed bag in the designated area or bins ready for refuse collection. If for any reason the bin liner punctures, put the damaged liner and waste inside a second bin liner. Wash out the inside of the swing bin itself with hot water and detergent.

Unused, leftover colour or lightener should be washed out of colouring bowls as soon as the stylist has finished the service. These products swell up if left for any length of time and therefore need to be washed away sooner rather than later, as they might increase the risk of blocking the drains.

TOP TIP

Barbicide is the routine way to keep combs hygienic throughout the day. Always rinse and dry items before they are used on clients.

ACTIVITY

Preventing contamination and cross-infection is an important aspect of general health and safety. Match the statements on the left with those on the right and write out the correct sentences.

Antibacterial Sprays Should be Used	For Total Sterilization of Styling Tools by Heat
An Autoclave is Used	For Sterilization by Penetrating Radiation
Barbicide is a Fluid Commonly Used	On Work Surfaces and Preparation Areas
Ultra-violet is	For Cleaning Sinks and Toilets
Household Bleach is an Effective Way	For Immersing Styling Tools Into

Antibacterial sprays should be used…	…for total sterilization of styling tools by heat.
An autoclave is used…	…for sterilization by penetrating radiation.
Barbicide is a fluid commonly used…	…on work surfaces and preparation areas.
Ultraviolet is…	…for cleaning sinks and toilets.
Household bleach is an effective way…	…for immersing styling tools in.

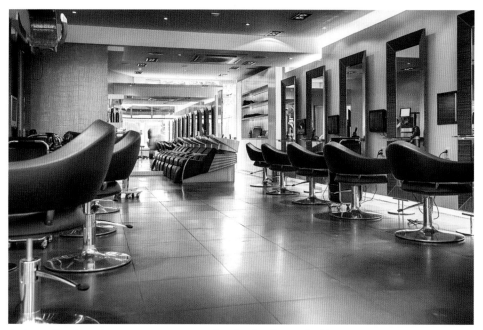

A clean, attractive salon conveys a message of professionalism and pride

TOP TIP

Different tools and items of equipment need to be sterilized in different ways. Plastic items such as combs, brushes and rollers cannot withstand the heat of an autoclave as they will lose their rigid properties and change shape as if they were melting. But a UV cabinet is very good for metal tools like scissors and plastic items.

HEALTH & SAFETY

Do not put contaminated items on work surfaces because they could spread infection.

ACTIVITY

Ask your supervisor what the arrangements are in your salon for the safe disposal of waste and sharps. Write your answers in your portfolio.

1. What are your salon's requirements for disposing of waste?

2. Are there any local bylaws affecting your salon and the way that it disposes of waste?

Daily salon maintenance

HEALTH & SAFETY

Electrical tools and equipment must have an annual portable appliance test (PAT) and be checked by a qualified person.

ACTIVITY

Copy and complete the table below in your portfolio by filling in the missing information.

Salon items	Where are they kept in your salon?	How are they stored in your salon?
Gowns and towels		
Heated styling equipment		
Salon styling products		
Retail stock items		
Basin/backwash products		
Colour materials		

Check and clean the salon equipment

Styling mirrors   Glass mirrors should always be sparkling clean! Clients sit in front of the mirrors for long periods so they will definitely see those murky smears. The mirrors need to be cleaned every morning before clients arrive and throughout the day using a window spray cleaner; this will quickly remove all the dirt, dust and hairspray.

Styling tools

ACTIVITY

Match the correct cleaner with the item it cleans and write out the correct pairs of letters and numbers.

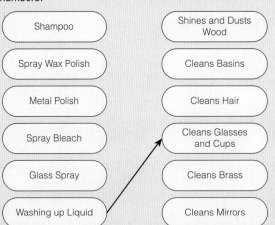

Shampoo	Shines and Dusts Wood
Spray Wax Polish	Cleans Basins
Metal Polish	Cleans Hair
Spray Bleach	Cleans Glasses and Cups
Glass Spray	Cleans Brass
Washing up Liquid	Cleans Mirrors

A.	Shampoo		1.	Shines and dusts wood
B.	Spray wax polish		2.	Cleans basins
C.	Metal polish		3.	Cleans hair
D.	Spray bleach		4.	Cleans glasses and cups
E.	Glass spray		5.	Cleans brass
F.	Washing up liquid		6.	Cleans mirrors

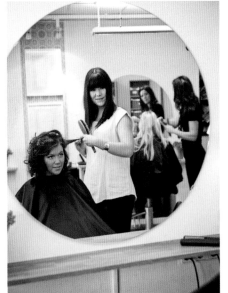

Clients will spot dirty, mucky or smeary marks on mirrors

For checking and cleaning styling tools refer back to the individual items covered earlier within this chapter.

Hood dryers, colour accelerators and steamers   Hood dryers, colour accelerators and steamers are made from tough vinyl mouldings over metal frames. They all run by electricity and should therefore be handled and cleaned with extreme care. Spray cleaners produce the best results because they expel the minimum amount of cleaning fluid, which helps to prevent product dripping into the equipment. This could cause it to malfunction or short-out.

Daily dusting and cleaning is done at the beginning and periodically throughout the day. When an item of equipment is used, say for a colour service, make sure that the equipment is checked and wiped immediately after use. This will ensure that other clients are not exposed to any hazards and that the machinery is clean and ready for use.

> For more information about hood dryers, colour accelerators and steamers refer back to the individual items covered earlier within this chapter.

Basin/backwash areas   Basins have ceramic finishes, which are hard-wearing but brittle. Never put metal, ceramic or glassware items into them because they could crack or be damaged. General cleaning should take place at the beginning of the day, although they will need routine checking and cleaning every time they are used. This is particularly important around the basin's neck area, especially after clients have had colouring or bleaching services. Simple spray cleaners containing bleach are an ideal, hygienic solution for both the bowl and chrome mixer valves as they minimize the possibility of cross-infection or cross-infestation.

Make sure that the **hair traps** are replaced regularly. These stop loose hairs going down drains and causing blockages, which could be both disruptive and expensive to put right.

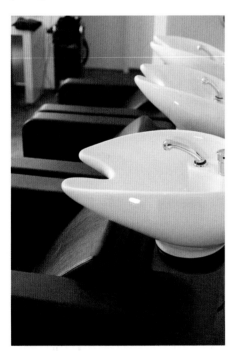

Basins need to be checked and cleaned after each use with spray bleach cleaner

TOP TIP

Always ask your supervisor what you can put down the basins. Never pour anything down the drain unless you know that it is safe.

HEALTH & SAFETY

Gowns should be machine washed to remove perfume, body odours or staining and to prevent the spread of cross-infection or cross-infestation.

Towels and gowns   Every client should have a clean, fresh towel and gown. These are an essential part of the daily salon equipment. Busy salons and barbers' shops tend to get through mountains of towels on a daily basis, so get to know how to use the salon's washing machine and tumble dryer. These will be in constant use and a quick, constant turnaround of laundry is expected.

Refilling and replenishing salon stock

Products need replacing on a daily basis. It is not good enough to leave things that need replacing for another day, or leave it for someone else to do. Without stock the other staff will not be able to use the correct products on their clients and potential sales will be lost.

At the basin The basins are in continual use, and as clients are shampooed and conditioned the products run down. Each type of shampoo and conditioner used by the salon at the backwash area is contained in large pump dispensers. When a product runs out, the correct product must be found from the stock room and refilled into the backwash size as soon as possible.

Carefully match the bulk sizes to the ones needing refilling. For each one, undo the screw top and clean the pump. Then, using a funnel, carefully top up the product to just below the neck. If you overfill you could waste product when you try to replace the pump. After filling the container, wipe up any spills and replace the bulk containers back into storage. You can then take the refills back to the basins.

Other products will be in continual use as stylists work on their clients. Keep checking up on salon styling materials so that they do not run out. If you notice that a product is getting low do not throw it away. Instead, ask the stylist if you should go and get a replacement out of stock ready for when it runs out.

In reception Retail displays in reception are an expensive investment for the salon and stock resting on shelves is an expensive cost. Products provide a useful income for the business and many shops and salons look for a significant proportion of their turnover from these sales.

Retail products will run down when clients buy them, so you can help the receptionist by keeping the stocks refilled throughout the day. You should ask permission to go and find the correct items so that the stock levels can be maintained. Always make a point of dusting the existing products on the shelf because people will not want to handle or buy dusty items. Retail displays should invite clients to browse; they prompt clients to ask questions or ask for advice.

Most hair products have a long shelf-life, so they will not perish or deteriorate over time like food products do. Nevertheless, as a routine way of selling older products first, it is normal practice to put the newer replacements at the back of the shelves and bring the older ones to the front. This system is called **stock rotation** and is a generally accepted practice.

Replace things after use

Equipment that is not put away can be a hazard. Each client deserves the best possible service and you can help by putting things away so that they are ready for next time. Hand dryers and heated equipment should be put back in their proper place for safety. Trailing leads need to be carefully coiled so that they do not present a hazard to the next user. Trolleys should be removed and their items cleaned and trays reorganized. Tools need to be cleaned and products put back tidily.

Clean working surfaces properly so that they are ready for use

Clean the work areas (reception, workstations, backwash and stock preparation areas). This means dusting and/or washing down at least once each day. Salons are designed with easy maintenance in mind so they have easy-to-wipe surfaces made of plastic, glass, tiles or lacquered wood.

When clients leave, the styling sections need to be made ready for use again. The styling sections are in continual use and no one wants to sit in someone else's hair clippings or left-behind debris. You need to clear the working surfaces of tools, cups and saucers, magazines, etc. The sections can be cleaned with spray surface cleaner or hot water and detergent; they are then dried and wiped free of smears so that they look shiny and appealing.

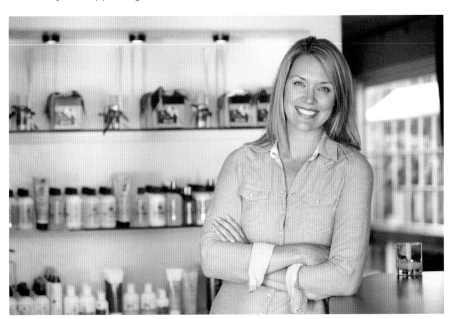

An eye-catching product display behind the salon reception desk will look attractive and entice clients to make a product purchase when they settle their payment.

> **TOP TIP**
>
> The barber's shop or hair salon is a public place and should always be clean and appealing. You have an important part to play in its overall success. Remember – a tidy salon is easier to clean so get into the habit of clearing work areas as you go along.

Daily salon maintenance (Continued...)

Salon floors and seating

The floors must be clean and clear of hazards at all times. This means that they will need regular mopping, sweeping or vacuuming, particularly following periods of wet weather when dirt is 'tracked in' from outside. When a work area is mopped, make sure that other staff (or clients) are aware that the area is wet and may be slippery. When using the vacuum cleaner, make a point of checking the collection bag and filters. It does not take long for hair clippings to fill the bag and this will prevent it from cleaning properly.

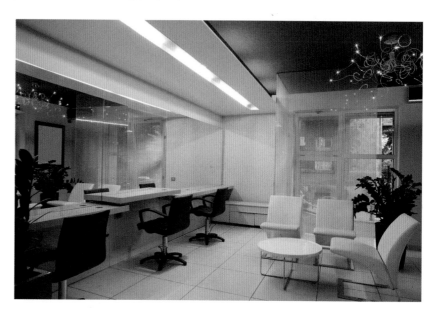

It is much easier to see that vinyl or ceramic floor coverings need cleaning than it is to see that a floor covered in carpet is dirty. If floors need mopping and cleaning, try to do this at a quieter time of the day, probably at the end of the working day so they can dry out overnight. If spillages happen during the day it will be necessary to mop up during times when clients are in the salon. When this occurs, make sure that any wet or damp areas are dried immediately afterwards because this will minimize the chance of anyone slipping.

ACTIVITY

Think about cleaning

Copy the table into your portfolio and fill in the missing information for how each item should be cleaned and how often it should be done.

Salon area	How should this be cleaned?	How often should it be done?
Work surfaces		
Glass and mirrors		
Carpets and working area floors		
Wash basins		

SUMMARY

Now you have finished this chapter you should have a clearer picture of everything relating to the tools and equipment that you will be using in the future. In particular, you should now have a basic understanding of:

✓ the wide variety of tools and equipment available and how they can be used

✓ how to maintain your equipment and optimize the lifespan of each item

✓ how to look after and maintain your modelling heads.

In addition, you will understand how this will help you to assist the hairdresser or barber.

REVISION QUESTIONS

Q1. Copy and complete this sentence: Clients should never be put at risk from cross-infection or cross- _____.

Fill in the blank

Q2. Sterilization kills all living organisms.

True or False

Q3. Which of the following should be sterilized in an autoclave? (You may choose more than one answer.)

brushes	☐	a
combs	☐	b
sectioning clips	☐	c
scissors	☐	d
clipper blades	☐	e
used razor blades	☐	f

Q4. Disinfectants kill all living organisms

True or False

Q5. Which of the following is a form of chemical sterilization? (Choose one answer.)

UV cabinet	○	a
autoclave	○	b
Barbicide™	○	c
disinfectant spray	○	d

3 Health and Safety in the Salon

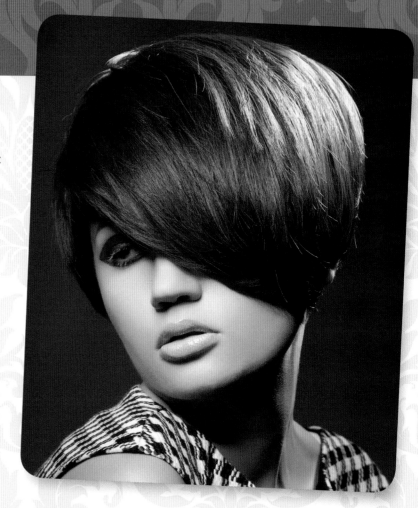

LEARNING OBJECTIVES

When you have finished this chapter you should:

◆ be able to spot hazards within the salon

◆ be able to work safely and hygienically at all times

◆ know your salon's emergency procedures

◆ understand how you can take care of your own personal hygiene

◆ know who you should report potential hazards to

◆ know your responsibilities under health and safety laws.

KEY TERMS

accident book

body odour

dermatitis

halitosis

HASAWA – Health and Safety at Work Act

hazard

legislation

risk

sharps box

sharps

sterilization

UV cabinet

INFORMATION COVERED IN THIS CHAPTER

PRACTICAL SKILLS

Look for potential hazards within the salon and take appropriate action to reduce risks.

Follow healthy and safe working practices at all times.

Tell other people about things that need attention or prompt action.

Be professional in your appearance and personal hygiene.

Be professional in your conduct at work.

Look for potential security risks whilst you are at work.

UNDERPINNING KNOWLEDGE

Know your salon's policy for healthy and safe working practices.

Understand your responsibilities under the Health and Safety at Work Act.

Know your salon's procedures for emergency evacuation and first aid.

Know how to work safely at all times.

Understand that other people may be affected by the things that you do in your work.

Understand the difference between hazard and risk.

INTRODUCTION

Health and safety is important for everyone working in the salon and it is vital that you understand the responsibility that you have for yourself and others – especially your colleagues and clients.

This chapter looks at the health and safety responsibilities you have at work, the way you go about your tasks and the impact or potential effect that your actions have on others in carrying out their work. Remember:

◆ Your actions should not create health and safety hazards.

◆ You should not ignore the hazards that could present a risk to others.

◆ You should take sensible, appropriate action to put things right; or

◆ You should tell someone immediately so that they can take the appropriate action.

Hazards and risk

Almost anything may be a **hazard**, but may or may not become a risk. Think about these examples:

◆ A trailing electric cable from a hairdryer is a hazard if it is trailing across a busy walkway through the salon, as there is a high risk of someone tripping over it, but if it lies along a wall or next to the work station out of the way, the risk is much less.

◆ Hydrogen peroxide is mixed with most colours and lighteners. It can be a serious chemical hazard and could present a high risk if left out in the salon. However, if it is kept in a locked COSHH cabinet and handled by properly trained people wearing personal protective equipment (PPE), the risk is much less.

◆ A failed light bulb could be a serious hazard in certain situations. If it is just one of many in a room, it presents very little risk, but if it is the only light on a stairwell it is a very high risk.

◆ A box of heavy material is a hazard. It presents a higher risk to someone who lifts it incorrectly, rather than someone who uses the correct manual handling techniques.

TOP TIP

Always wear disposable polyvinyl or nitrile gloves when handling chemicals.

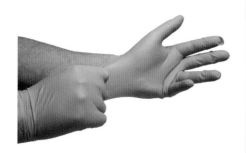

ACTIVITY

Think about some of the hazards that could exist in your workplace. Copy the table below and fill in the missing information.

Potential hazard	Why is this a hazard in the salon/barber's shop?	How could this risk be reduced?
Loose carpet edge in reception		
Boxes stacked up in the fire escape		
Water spilt on the floor near the basins		
Hair clippings left on the salon floor		
Loose plug on a blow-dryer		
A stylist drops their comb on the floor, picks it up and then uses it on a client		

HEALTH & SAFETY

If you would like to find out more about hairdressing health and safety or the relevant legislation covered in the (HASAWA) Health and Safety at Work Act (1974), go online to the Health and Safety Executive HSE website: www.hse.gov.uk/hairdressing

Hazards can be related to all aspects of work. Here are a few examples around the salon:

1 Hazards to do with the working **environment**:

◆ wet or slippery floors

◆ cluttered passageways or corridors

◆ hair clippings left on the salon floor

◆ trailing electrical flexes

2 Hazards to do with **equipment and materials**:

◆ worn or faulty electrical equipment

◆ incorrectly labelled materials

◆ mishandling or inaccurate measurement of chemicals

3 Hazards connected with **people**:

◆ bad posture

◆ poor health, cross-infection, disease

◆ handling and moving stock

Working with electricity

Electricity can kill. Although deaths from electric shocks are very rare in hairdressing salons, even a non-fatal shock can cause severe and permanent injury. An electric shock from faulty or damaged electrical equipment may lead to a fall, for example down a stairwell.

Those using electricity may not be the only ones at risk. Poor electrical installations and faulty electrical appliances can lead to fires, which can also result in death or injury to others.

Get into the habit of looking for loose cables and plugs on tongs, straighteners and hairdryers before plugging them in for use. If you think that a piece of electrical equipment is faulty or damaged, tell your supervisor immediately and they will label it, making sure that no one else tries to use it.

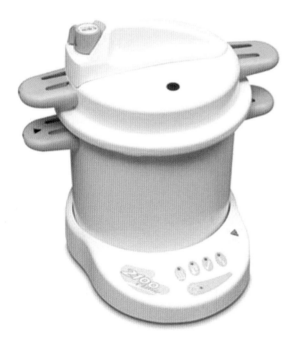

The autoclave sterilizes tools and equipment by using heat

TOP TIP

Up to 70 per cent of hairdressers suffer from work-related skin damage such as dermatitis at some point during their career. Most cases are preventable.

TOP TIP

Health and safety information is everywhere; there will be posters and signs explaining a range of things, like how to find and use fire equipment, where you should go if there is an emergency and how to handle the products safely.

For more information on working with electricity, see Electricity at Work Regulations 1989 in Appendix 1.

TOP TIP

Never use an autoclave to sterilize a stylist's scissors, they may damage the precision surfaces.

Thinking about your work routines

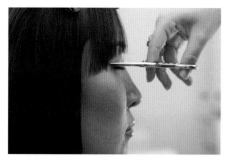

Precision cutting requires total concentration

Because you work in public service, *all* of your day-to-day routines will have some form of impact on someone. You must be aware of things that could harm yourself or other people. You must stay alert at all times when you are working.

From a legal point of view, you are bound by law under the **Health and Safety at Work Act HASAWA** 1974 to have a duty of care, not only to yourself, but also to anyone else who could be affected by your actions. Your physical wellbeing is vitally important. Too many late nights and over-indulgences or added stress from personal issues will affect the way that you carry out your duties. Any lapses in your concentration can have a disastrous impact on you, your client or anyone else in the salon.

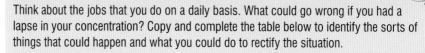

ACTIVITY

Think about the jobs that you do on a daily basis. What could go wrong if you had a lapse in your concentration? Copy and complete the table below to identify the sorts of things that could happen and what you could do to rectify the situation.

Area of work	What could go wrong?	What should you do?
Applying a neutralizer to curlers on a client		
Taking a colour off at the basin		
Mixing up a colour for a stylist, but using the wrong hydrogen peroxide concentration		
Moving a large delivery of stock from reception to the stock room		
Preparing a styling unit with equipment for a stylist, but a lead is loose on a hairdryer		

HEALTH & SAFETY

Employers have a responsibility to ensure the health, safety and welfare of the people within the workplace. All people at work have a duty and responsibility not to harm themselves or others through the work they do.

TOP TIP

It is very important that you understand the terms 'hazard', 'risk' and 'control'. The Health and Safety Executive (HSE) is the body appointed to support and enforce health and safety law and they have defined these terms as follows:

◆ Hazard: something with potential to cause harm.
◆ Risk: the likelihood of the hazard's potential being realized.
◆ Control: the means by which risks identified are eliminated or reduced to acceptable levels.

Being responsible

Simply being aware of potential hazards is not enough; you have a responsibility to make the salon a safe working environment for everyone. Suppose, for example, that someone had carelessly blocked a fire door with a stock delivery. You could handle this yourself by moving the items of stock to a safe and secure location.

You will be able to deal with some hazards but not others; you will have to consider each one carefully before you do anything. Remember, if you are not sure, ask a senior colleague.

Here are some examples of hazards that you could deal with yourself:

◆ trailing leads/flexes – roll them up and store them safely

◆ cluttered doorways and corridors – remove objects and store them safely or dispose of them appropriately

◆ hair clippings on the floor – sweep them up.

These are hazards that you should report to your manager:

◆ faulty equipment such as hairdryers, tongs, straightening irons, kettles, computers, etc.

◆ worn floor coverings or broken tiles

◆ loose or damaged fittings, such as mirrors, shelves or back washes

◆ obstructions that are too heavy for you to move safely.

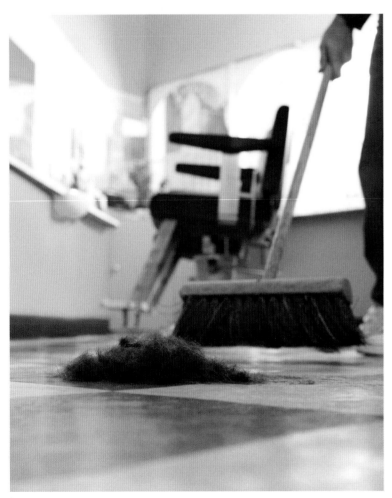

Loose clippings are a hazard to everyone walking around the salon as people could slip on them. Make sure that they are swept up promptly and put in the bin.

A safe and healthy working environment

ACTIVITY

Salon layout

Draw a floor plan of your salon. Show where the following can be found:

- fire extinguisher(s)
- storage for products/equipment
- disposal of waste and sharps
- sterilizing equipment
- personal protective equipment (PPE)
- accident book
- fire exit(s)
- first aid box/kit
- health and safety information
- assembly point

The **Health and Safety at Work Act (HASAWA) 1974** is the main, overarching legislation, made by parliament. This Act contains many individual regulations and the responsibility for maintaining these falls upon you and your employer.

An employer has a legal duty to ensure that:

- the premises are safe to work within
- all equipment and salon systems are safe to use
- employees have access to personal protective equipment
- health and safety systems are appropriately reviewed and updated
- staff are trained so they can do their duties safely.

The employees have a legal duty to:

- follow appropriate systems of work laid down for their safety
- make proper use of equipment provided for their safety
- co-operate with their employer on health and safety matters
- inform their employer if they identify hazardous activities/situations
- take care to ensure that their activities do not put others at risk.

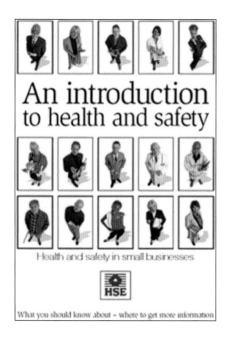

An introduction to health and safety

Health and safety in small businesses

HSE

What you should know about – where to get more information

For more specific information on individual health and safety regulations, see Appendix 1.

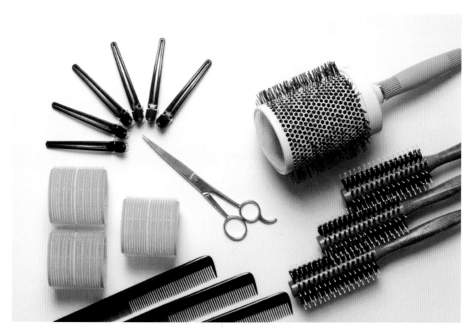

Organise your tools and equipment and keep them clean and hygienic, ready for use

ACTIVITY

The Health and Safety at Work Act 1974 is continually being reviewed and updated. It covers many smaller component regulations. Match the individual legal regulations on the left with the appropriate health and safety issues on the right and write out the correct pairs. (Hint: look at the regulation wording to work out its appropriate link.)

A	Workplace (Health, Safety and Welfare) Regulations 1992	1	Always wear gloves and aprons when handling chemical compounds
B	Manual Handling Operations Regulations 1992	2	Correct and safe operation of salon equipment
C	Provision and Use of Work Equipment Regulations (PUWER) 1998	3	Salon chemical products must be kept safely stored away at all times
D	Personal Protective Equipment at Work Regulations 1992	4	Dermatitis is a notifiable skin condition that results from sensitivity to chemicals
E	Control of Substances Hazardous to Health (COSHH) Regulations 2002	5	Monitoring and maintenance of workplace hygiene and cleanliness
F	Electricity at Work Regulations 1989	6	Always keep well stocked in case of accidents occurring at work
G	Reporting of Injuries, Diseases and Dangerous Occurrences Regulations (RIDDOR) 1995	7	Manufacturers' information relating to the use of chemical products
H	Cosmetic Products (Safety) Regulations 1989	8	The movement and handling of objects needs to be carried out safely and properly
I	Health and Safety (First Aid) Regulations 1981	9	Items of salon electrical equipment must be checked and tested once a year

TOP TIP

We all have a duty to safeguard our environment. Be environmentally aware when you dispose of waste.

BEST PRACTICE

If you use chemicals such as permanent wave lotions or colouring products, always wear disposable gloves. Not only will this protect your skin from chemical hazards, it will also stop your hands from becoming stained, which looks unprofessional.

Disposal of waste

General waste Most salon waste is harmless and as long as it has been sorted for recycling it can be put out for normal commercial rubbish collection.

Non-food waste items such as empty polythene containers, cotton wool and plastic caps are not recyclable so should be put into bin liners. When they are almost full, the liners can be removed and sealed by tying in a knot. The empty bin should be washed with detergent, dried and a new bin liner installed.

Being environmentally aware means being more responsible in how we dispose of our waste items. Different local authorities have specific arrangements for safe disposal and recycling. Some items should be cleared away promptly. For example, simple hair clippings left on the salon floor are a potential hazard. Although hair itself is not hazardous waste, it becomes a risk to health and safety if left on the salon floor.

Disposal of sharp items Sharp items such as disposable razor blades need to be handled with extreme care. Used **sharps** (the term used to describe them) must be disposed of carefully to prevent any injury or cross-infection. Razor blades and similar items should be placed into a **sharps box** – a safe, sealed container. When the container is full, it can be disposed of safely. This type of salon waste should be kept away from general salon waste as special arrangements for its disposal may be provided by your local authority.

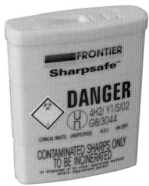

Use a sharps bin to dispose of all sharp items such as razor blades

A safe and healthy working environment (Continued...)

Lifting and handling

Bad posture and incorrect handling of large and/or heavy items can result in lower back pain, other back problems and strain disorders. You must always take care if you need to move anything. Think about the situations that can occur in a salon environment, for example:

- moving stock into storage
- unpacking heavy or awkward items
- lifting equipment and moving salon furniture.

For more information on the Manual Handling Operations Regulations 1992, see Appendix 1.

Avoiding dermatitis

The Health and Safety Executive (HSE) conducted a survey across the industry and found that almost 70 per cent of people who start hairdressing and barbering develop a condition called **dermatitis**. This is a painful condition caused by failing to wear disposable polyvinyl or nitrile gloves during shampoo and conditioning. Many people who develop this condition have to stop hairdressing, so this is a serious occupational health hazard. Always dry your hands thoroughly after immersing them in water and apply moisturizer to keep the skin hydrated.

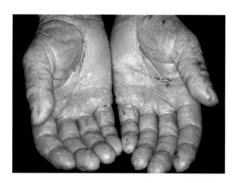

Five steps to preventing dermatitis

1. Wear disposable polyvinyl/nitrile gloves when rinsing, shampooing, colouring, lightening, etc.
2. Dry your hands thoroughly with a soft cotton or paper towel.
3. Moisturize after washing your hands, as well as at the start and end of each day. Be thorough – it is easy to miss between the fingers, your fingertips or wrists.
4. Change gloves between clients. Make sure you do not contaminate your hands when you take them off.
5. Check the skin regularly for early signs of dermatitis.

What do you do if you think you have dermatitis?   If you think you are suffering from dermatitis, visit your doctor for advice and treatment. If you think it has been caused or made worse by your work, mention this to your doctor and tell your employer.

Handling chemicals

Many hairdressing services involve some contact with chemicals. You must always follow the product manufacturer's instructions for their safe use and application. Chemicals include perming lotions, neutralizers, colouring products and hydrogen peroxide. These are hazardous and present a high risk to anyone who does not know

ACTIVITY

Find out the following information from your place of work and keep a record in your portfolio for future reference.

1. Who has overall responsibility for health and safety?
2. What is this person's role in the workplace?
3. If you found something that you felt was not safe at work, who would you report to?
4. What sort of unsafe things do you think you might find? (List as many as you can.)
5. In relation to product use, why are manufacturers' instructions important?
6. What is the salon's policy in respect to maintaining a healthy and safe work environment?

the correct procedures for their use. They must be handled, stored, used and disposed of correctly in accordance with the Control of Substances Hazardous to Health Regulations (2003), also known as the 'COSHH Regulations'.

COSHH precautions Your employer will have carried out a risk assessment for all the products that you use within the salon. This risk assessment covers everything that you use and provides guidance for the safe ways in which they may be handled. The list of chemical products will vary from cleaning items such as washing materials, bleach and polish, to the more typical salon specific items such as colours, lighteners, hydrogen peroxide and general styling materials.

The risk assessment will show:

◆ a hazard rating for each product listed – the level of risk that each of the chemical products presents to you;

◆ details on how they can be handled safely with the use of personal protective equipment (PPE).

> **BEST PRACTICE**
>
> Health and safety laws are being continually reviewed and updated. Make sure you are aware of the latest information and look at the health and safety posters within your salon.

Personal protective equipment (PPE)

Your employer will provide PPE for you and your clients. Your protective equipment will typically be disposable gloves and plastic aprons. You *must* wear these items whenever you are handling chemicals. Watch the stylists to see the times when and the reasons why they wear these items. The PPE for clients are gowns, towels and plastic capes. Clients should wear the sleeved type styling gowns in the salon for all chemical processes such as colouring, lightening and perming, and will often wear them for cutting and styling too. However, a sleeveless cutting square is perfectly acceptable for cutting only services.

A clean, fresh towel is used to protect the client and their clothes from becoming wet during shampooing, or at any service provided at the basin. They also sit with a towel fastened around their shoulders when they are waiting. In addition to towels, salons provide plastic capes that are worn over the top of towels to protect them from staining, and the clients from chemical spills or staining.

> **TOP TIP**
>
> Up to 70 per cent of hairdressers suffer from skin damage. Keep your hands healthy and avoid 'bad hand days'. Moisturize regularly and always wear disposable non-latex gloves when you handle any chemical products.

ACTIVITY

Copy and complete the table below by filling in the missing information.

Type of PPE	When is it used?	Why is it used?
Disposable non-latex gloves		
Gowns and towels		
Stylist's waterproof apron		
Barrier cream		
Cotton wool		

See Appendix 1 for more information on the Personal Protective Equipment at Work Regulations 1992.

A safe and healthy working environment (Continued...)

Slips and trips

The most common cause of injuries at work is the slip or trip. Falls can be serious and a busy salon means lots of people, and the more clients there are the more hair clippings there will be. Loose clippings left on the salon floor present a hazard to staff and clients alike. Both wet and dry hair clippings are easily slipped on, so make sure that you sweep the working areas regularly. Don't wait for stylists to finish – get rid of clippings before they build up. Clear them away from areas where people are working or walking and put them into the waste bin. Wet floors are also a hazard within the salon, particularly in busy traffic thoroughfares. Any spillages need to be cleared up immediately.

Look out for trailing leads. Portable electrical items such as hairdryers, tongs and straighteners plugged in at the styling unit can be a hazard to everyone as it is very easy to trip on the lead.

TOP TIP

Always check for these hazards:

◆ Floors – are they slippery or wet?

◆ Doorways – are they clear of obstacles?

◆ Electrical flexes – are they loose or trailing?

◆ Chemicals – are they labelled and stored correctly?

◆ Equipment – is it worn or in need of attention?

Spillages and breakages

If something gets spilled or broken you need to act quickly, but stop and think before doing anything. Ask yourself these questions:

◆ What has been spilled or dropped?

◆ Is this something that needs special care and attention when handling?

◆ Should you report the situation to someone else, or can you handle the situation yourself?

◆ If you can, should you be wearing gloves?

TOP TIP

If you are not sure about something, ask someone in authority.

ACTIVITY

What would you do if you found the following hazards? Copy and complete the table, putting a tick in the appropriate box for each hazard. Ask your supervisor to check it when you have finished.

Hazard	Sort it out myself	Report it
Unsafe stacking of boxes in the stock room		
Faulty kettle in the kitchen		
Failed light bulb in the corridor		
Spillage on the salon floor		
A broken glass in the kitchen		
Smoke appearing around the door of a closed room		
Bare cable showing on the flex of a hand dryer		
Supervisor's signature:	**Date:**	

Preventing infection

A warm, humid salon can offer a perfect home for disease-carrying bacteria. If they can find food in the form of dust and dirt they may reproduce rapidly. Good ventilation, however, provides a circulating air current that will help to prevent their growth. This is why it is important to keep the salon clean, dry and well aired at all times. This includes clothing, work areas, tools and all equipment.

Head lice and nits

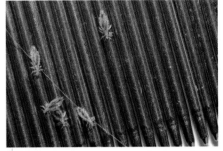

Removal of nits using a fine-tooth nit-comb

This extremely common infestation can be very difficult to stop, particularly among young school children. Head lice are minute animal parasites that feed on the host's blood. The infection can be observed in either the egg stage or the 'adult' head louse stage, depending on how long the client has been infected. Head lice are passed from person to person through direct contact, and infestation is always accompanied by itching (caused by the parasite biting the scalp to feed on the host's blood). The adult louse lays eggs (called nits) and cements these to individual hairs close to the scalp. The incubation period is short and within days, an immature louse emerges.

A number of products to combat head lice can be obtained from the chemist or, alternatively, from natural remedy sources and herbalists. Getting rid of the adult parasite is easy, but it is much more difficult to destroy the nits. After an infected person has been treated with the shampoo or lotion, the nits need to be removed to break the head louse life cycle. The easiest way to remove the nits is to use a fine-tooth nit-comb when the hair is still wet. Applying vinegar (a mild acid solution) to the hair tightens the hair cuticle layer and makes it easier to comb away the nits. A final shampoo will remove any unpleasant smell and the hair is then free from infestation.

Sterilization

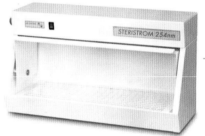

A UV radiation sterilizing cabinet

Sterilization is the most effective way of providing hygienically safe tools to work with in salons. Sterilization means the complete eradication of living organisms.

Ultraviolet radiation
Ultraviolet (UV) radiation cabinets are a typical method for sterilizing tools and equipment in the salon or barber shop.

Chemical sterilizers
Chemical sterilizers should be handled only with suitable PPE, as many of the solutions used are hazardous to health and should not come into contact with the skin. The most effective form of salon sterilization is achieved by the total immersion of the contaminated implements into a jar of fluid.

Autoclave
The autoclave provides a very efficient way of sterilizing using heat. It is particularly good for metal tools, although the high temperatures are not suitable for plastics such as brushes and combs. Items placed in the autoclave take around 20 minutes to sterilize. (Check with manufacturers' instructions for variations.)

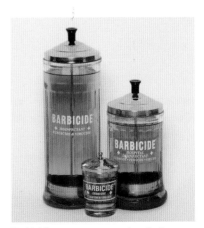

Barbicide™ – a common chemical disinfectant in the salon

Risks to health and safety

Emergencies: fire

There are situations such as fire, where the building must be evacuated immediately and everyone needs to be informed so that staff and clients can make their way to the designated assembly point(s).

All places of work must have adequate firefighting equipment and means of escape. All fire exits have to be clearly marked with the appropriate signs and it must be possible to open all doors easily and immediately from the inside.

Fire can occur in many situations:

- electrical faults – faulty wiring, overloading power sockets with multi-way adapters
- badly maintained equipment within the salon or staff only areas
- gas appliances left unattended
- badly positioned portable heaters – bottle gas space heaters, electric convector or fan heaters.

It is important to learn the evacuation process and practise it regularly. You need to know where the exits from the building are and where you need to regroup outside the building.

General evacuation rules
If a fire breaks out in the salon, the first thing that should be done is to raise the alarm. The person who discovers the fire should immediately tell the person in charge, who will then organize the evacuation. Staff should take responsibility for assisting clients to evacuate safely. No one should stop to collect anything. Staff and clients should assemble at the assembly point and a senior member of staff should check that everyone is accounted for.

A member of staff should call the fire brigade by dialling 999. If you have to do this then you will need to make sure that you have the right information ready to give the operator. You should never try and fight the fire yourself unless you have been properly trained to use the equipment and it is safe to do so. If it is safe to do so, all windows and doors should be closed, as this will slow down the progress of the fire.

Firefighting equipment
Firefighting equipment must be available and located in specific areas. The equipment should only be used by properly trained people and only when it is safe to do so. It is very important that the right equipment is used. Using the wrong equipment could make the fire worse and endanger the person using it.

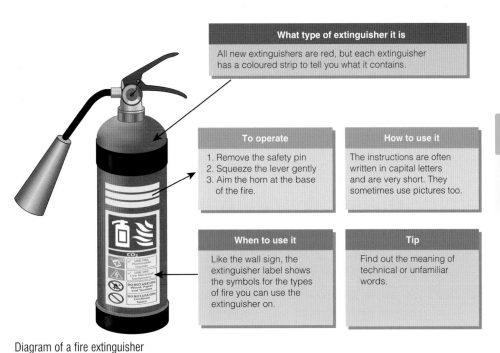

What type of extinguisher it is

All new extinguishers are red, but each extinguisher has a coloured strip to tell you what it contains.

To operate

1. Remove the safety pin
2. Squeeze the lever gently
3. Aim the horn at the base of the fire.

How to use it

The instructions are often written in capital letters and are very short. They sometimes use pictures too.

When to use it

Like the wall sign, the extinguisher label shows the symbols for the types of fire you can use the extinguisher on.

Tip

Find out the meaning of technical or unfamiliar words.

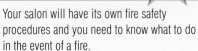

BEST PRACTICE

Your salon will have its own fire safety procedures and you need to know what to do in the event of a fire.

Diagram of a fire extinguisher

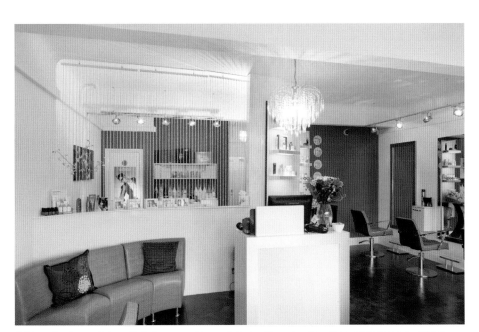

A tidy salon is much less likely to present hazards to health and safety. Take pride in your working environment and it will be a place where you enjoy working and your clients feel relaxed.

Risks to health and safety (Continued...)

Different types of fire extinguishers are used to fight different types of fire and they are colour coded according to type. You must recognize these different types of fire extinguisher and be able to classify the type of fire in order to select the right type of firefighting equipment.

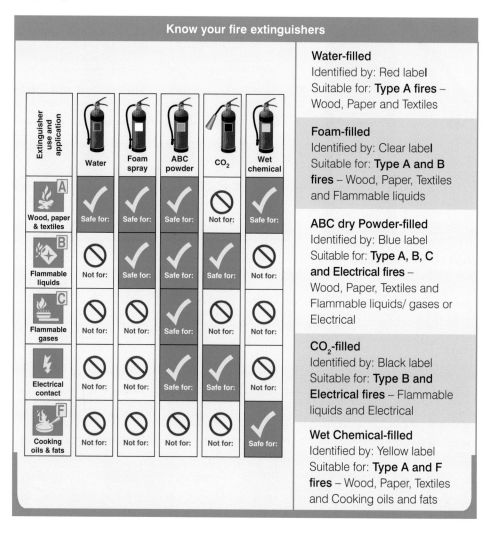

Know your fire extinguishers

Water-filled
Identified by: Red label
Suitable for: **Type A fires** – Wood, Paper and Textiles

Foam-filled
Identified by: Clear label
Suitable for: **Type A and B fires** – Wood, Paper, Textiles and Flammable liquids

ABC dry Powder-filled
Identified by: Blue label
Suitable for: **Type A, B, C and Electrical fires** – Wood, Paper, Textiles and Flammable liquids/ gases or Electrical

CO_2-filled
Identified by: Black label
Suitable for: **Type B and Electrical fires** – Flammable liquids and Electrical

Wet Chemical-filled
Identified by: Yellow label
Suitable for: **Type A and F fires** – Wood, Paper, Textiles and Cooking oils and fats

Accidents can be caused by any of the following:

◆ carelessness
◆ inappropriate behaviour
◆ tiredness
◆ misuse of substances (drink or drugs)
◆ faulty equipment
◆ poorly stored chemicals
◆ untidy and dirty work area
◆ poor salon layout.

The salon must have a first aid box that is correctly stocked with all the necessary items needed to deal with minor accidents. The regulations also cover the need to provide qualified first aiders.

ACTIVITY

Fire knowledge quiz

Write the letter of the correct answer for questions 1 to 3.

1   What is the main colour of a fire exit sign?

   A. green

   B. blue

   C. red

   D. yellow

2   What should you do first when you hear a fire alarm?

   A. phone the fire brigade

   B. evacuate the building

   C. check to see where the fire is

   D. wait in the staff room

3   What colour are fire extinguishers?

   A. red

   B. green

   C. black

   D. blue

4   Water-filled extinguishers can be used on electrical fires: true or false?

5   Fire exits must always be kept locked: true or false?

ACTIVITY

Fill in the missing information.

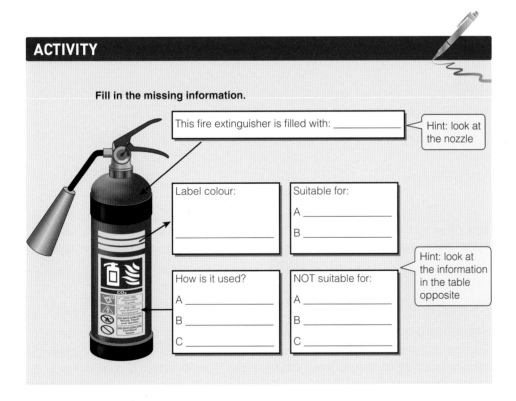

This fire extinguisher is filled with: _____

Hint: look at the nozzle

Label colour:

_____

Suitable for:

A _____

B _____

Hint: look at the information in the table opposite

How is it used?

A _____

B _____

C _____

NOT suitable for:

A _____

B _____

C _____

Accidents

Accidents can occur at any time and most of the time these will not be too serious. However, all accidents must be recorded in an **accident book** that must be kept in the salon. It should contain all the details of the accident, who was involved, how it happened, what action was taken, details of any witnesses, etc.

Dressing and behaving professionally

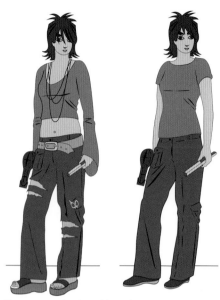

You must maintain a tidy and professional appearance at all times

Personal appearance

The effort we put into getting ready for work reflects our pride in our work and that we care about what we do. Sometimes we have to wear things that we would not wear if we had a personal choice, but professional standards and salon image must come first.

Clothes   Workwear should be practical and easy to maintain. Clothes should be easy to clean and iron if necessary and made of suitable fabrics. They should not be tight and restrictive, which would make working harder and more tiring; they may also make you perspire and increase body odour (BO).

Shoes   Hairdressers and barbers should wear flat or low-heeled shoes that enclose the feet (cover the toes). We spend most of our time on our feet so comfortable shoes will help prevent backache.

Hair   As hair professionals, our hair is an advertisement for our skill in the salon. If your hair is a mess, think about how that will affect your clients' confidence in you. Your hair should always look good and well-styled to reflect the salon image. Your hair should always be clean, tidy and representative of the place where you work.

Make-up   If you wear make-up to work, make sure that you check with your salon supervisor to see what is acceptable and appropriate.

Nails   You should have similar length, short, neatly manicured nails. Polish can be worn but must not be chipped or badly applied.

Jewellery   Wear only a minimum of jewellery while you are working. It can harbour germs and it can be uncomfortable for the client because it can get tangled in their hair.

TOP TIP

First impressions are lasting impressions; you do not get a second chance to create a good first impression.

BEST PRACTICE

In some salons and barber shops you will find that a professional uniform will be the appropriate, permitted dress code. Other salons and shops have a dress code but on a less formal basis. You will know what is required and acceptable at your place of work from what is stated in your induction. Regardless of dress code, you will always need to turn up for work in clean, ironed clothing.

Personal health, hygiene and behaviour

Hands and nails   Make sure your hands are very clean. Dirty hands are not only unattractive, but also spread germs and could cross-infect your clients. Your hands are very important; they are the way you earn a living, so they need to be carefully looked after. Keep your nails clean, especially underneath, and try to keep them neatly manicured and not too long. Check them regularly for any disorders.

Always wash your hands before work, after using the toilet and after coughing or sneezing. This will reduce the risk of spreading infections to others. Use moisturizing creams regularly to help replace the moisture lost by constant washing. When you shampoo, for example, it may be helpful to apply a moisturizing cream. If the skin on your hands is allowed to become dry, it will crack and become very sore. This may prevent you from working until it heals.

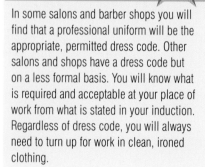

Some people may suffer from dermatitis from exposure to all the chemicals used in the profession. If your hands continue to be sore and do not heal, consult your doctor. In some cases, a person's sensitivity could mean that they have to give up their job.

Body   The body has sweat glands all over its surface that are used to help control the body temperature by secreting moisture out on to the surface of the skin when you are hot. This provides a good breeding ground for bacteria, which in turn causes body odour (BO). It is essential that you have a shower or bath at least every day and use deodorants, antiperspirants or similar.

Mouth   Unpleasant breath (halitosis) can be offensive to others. It can be caused by all sorts of things we have eaten, like onions or garlic, which are usually temporary; by smoking; stomach upsets; or other problems, such as pieces of food that get stuck between the teeth and then decay. As you will be working very close to the client, you will be breathing very close to them and so they will be able to smell any bad breath easily. Do not smoke at all when you are on duty.

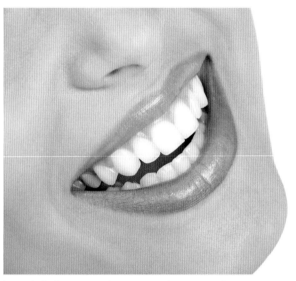

In our industry, personal appearance is paramount

Feet   Like our hands, our feet are important because we do most of our work standing. We have looked at the sort of shoes we wear and must make sure they fit properly. You should also wash your feet regularly – some people's feet sweat a lot and this can cause foot odour. Make sure minor problems like verrucas, corns and athlete's foot are treated. Some disorders of the feet can make standing painful so you need to get them treated as soon as possible. Keep your toenails short: they should be cut and filed regularly so that they do not become painful during long periods of standing during the day.

BEST PRACTICE

Bad breath can easily be offensive to other people. To prevent bad breath brush your teeth regularly, particularly after eating, have regular dental checks and use a mouthwash or breath freshener. Dental type chewing gums work very well but may not be appropriate in the salon; always check with your salon supervisor first. Do not smoke when you're on duty.

TOP TIP

Always check your appearance before you start work, and do not forget to recheck throughout the day.

TOP TIP

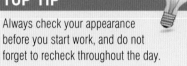

Coping with the stresses of hairdressing and barbering, which at times can be serious, is another thing we must learn to do.

Personal well-being

To work successfully as a hairdresser or a barber, you will need energy and stamina. Having a good health routine will give you that energy and stamina. The first aspect of that routine would be a well-balanced diet, one that is healthy and nutritious. You should take regular exercise; perhaps try playing sport or dancing. You should also get sufficient sleep and relaxation to help you recover from the stresses of the working day (it is often recommended that we have eight hours of sleep a day).

Good posture is necessary – as hair professionals we have to stand for long periods. Correct posture by standing properly will help prevent backache and, in the long term, back problems and other conditions like varicose veins. Always stand with the back straight, your feet apart and your weight evenly distributed on both legs. Do not stand with all your weight on one leg and your pelvis tilted. If you stand like this for long periods you will get backache and possibly more serious problems with your lower back; you will also increase the risk of developing varicose veins.

The care and attention you pay to how you present yourself for work is very important to your success and progress. Whatever job you do, make sure you look the part. Being thorough about your personal hygiene will ensure that you do not cause offence to anyone else, either to your clients or your colleagues. It can be embarrassing to be told you have a hygiene problem; the best way to avoid this is to make sure you do not have to be told.

Personal behaviour

The salon or barber's shop is a professional environment and you are on show. The way that you react to others and the respect that you show will be apparent by not only what you say, but also how you say it. Treat others with a mutual, professional respect – regardless of what you think or would like to say. Always conduct your work in a safe, professional manner; never fool around, as this could put others at risk by your actions or negligence.

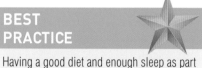

BEST PRACTICE

Having a good diet and enough sleep as part of a good health routine will make sure that you can always give your best to the clients, your colleagues and your employer.

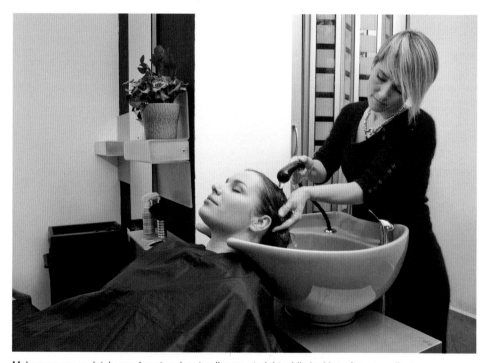

Make sure you maintain good posture by standing up straight while looking after your client

SUMMARY

Now you have finished this chapter you should have a clearer picture of all the essential aspects associated with working safely within the salon. In particular, you should now have a basic understanding of:

✓ working safely and preventing the risk of injury to yourself or others

✓ identifying hazards and risks to health and safety

✓ taking appropriate action in order to reduce the hazards affecting other people

✓ preventing the spread of infection and diseases to other people within the salon

✓ taking care of yourself and your own well-being

✓ knowing how to respond in the event of an emergency.

In addition, you will understand how these principles will enable you to work confidently but safely at all times.

REVISION QUESTIONS

Q1. Copy and complete this sentence: A hazard is something with a potential to cause _____.

Fill in the blank

Q2. Risk is the likelihood of the hazard's potential being realized?

True or false?

Q3. Which of the following are examples of hazards in the workplace? (You may choose more than one answer.)

hair clippings on the floor	☐ a
plugged-in appliances	☐ b
trailing flexes across thoroughfares	☐ c
products on retail shelves	☐ d
difficult clients	☐ e
blocked fire doors	☐ f

Q4. If a comb is dropped on the floor during use, it should be sterilized before it is used again?

True or false?

Q5. Which of the following is considered to be an occupational health hazard? (Choose one answer.)

head lice	○ a
nits	○ b
split ends	○ c
dermatitis	○ d

4 Working Together

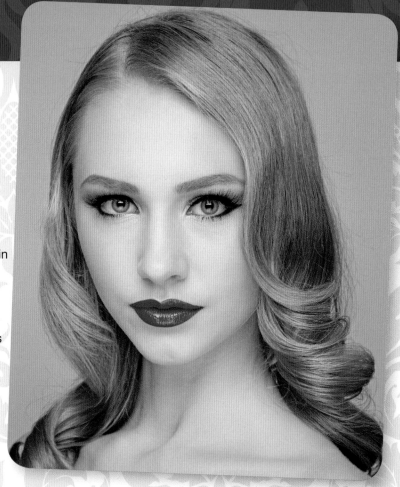

LEARNING OBJECTIVES

When you have finished this chapter you should:

◆ be able to work as part of a team

◆ be able to develop and maintain a professional relationship with clients and colleagues

◆ be able to develop your own skills and abilities in your work

◆ know how to improve and work towards targets

◆ know your salon's policies and legal obligations

◆ be able to communicate professionally and provide aftercare advice.

KEY TERMS

appraisal

body language

empathy

jargon

goodwill

personal development plan

INFORMATION COVERED IN THIS CHAPTER

PRACTICAL SKILLS

Be able to help and support your colleagues.

Be able to help and provide information to the salon's clients.

Be able to communicate professionally.

Be able to find ways to improve your own performance.

Be able to work towards personal targets.

Make sure that you update the client's records after consultation.

UNDERPINNING KNOWLEDGE

Know how to work with others in harmony.

Know how to communicate effectively and professionally.

Understand the salon's policies and rules.

Know how to find ways to develop your own skills and knowledge in your work.

Know who can help and support you in developing yourself in your work.

INTRODUCTION

Clients are the most important people in the salon, and without them there would not be a salon to work in. Therefore:

◆ We must create and maintain a professional approach to service which is customer-focused. That means putting the clients and their goodwill first, even if it means putting ourselves last.

◆ We must work with our colleagues in ways that support them in doing what they need to do, and treat them with courtesy and respect so that there is never an atmosphere or any unpleasantness.

Quite simply, we want the salon's clients to feel welcome when they enter the salon and enjoy the experience throughout the service. That way, we know that we have done everything possible to make them feel special, and we can expect them to come back on a regular basis.

Building professional relationships

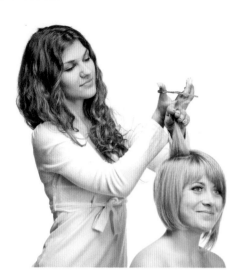

When we meet someone for the first time we often make judgements about what they are like and usually for all the wrong reasons. For example, we make judgements based on:

◆ the way people look

◆ their age

◆ the way they speak

◆ the way that they move around.

For these reasons it is very important to make a good first impression.

We can influence other people's views by:

◆ the courtesy and politeness that we show

◆ the genuine interest that we have for them

◆ our **body language**

◆ the way that we talk to them, or the way that we respond to their needs.

Put simply, it is all about communication.

Signs of good communication

The signs of good communication are:

◆ listening and responding to the clients' requests

◆ treating people with respect

◆ being confident, polite and courteous

◆ positive body language

◆ supporting the clients by asking if they need anything.

Listening and responding to the clients' requests   You can show that you are listening to the clients by acting upon the information they give you. Let them finish what they are saying before you respond; never try to guess what they want or need – you may feel foolish if you get it wrong.

Treating people with respect   Always treat clients with respect. People want and deserve to feel valued and you can do this by treating them in the same way that you would wish to be treated yourself. Try putting yourself in other people's situations and see things from their point of view. This is a special skill called **empathy**, and not everyone possesses this ability.

Being confident, polite and courteous   Communicate clearly and confidently with clients at all times. The clients are usually genuinely interested in you and your contribution to the overall salon team. They will be impressed by your ability to talk confidently and comfortably about things that interest you. Try to remember that although confidence is important, being polite and courteous shows that you are interested in their well-being too. Always speak in a friendly way to clients and colleagues.

BEST PRACTICE

Give clients the time to tell you what they want. Do not try to double-guess them or try to anticipate their needs. You may be considered uncaring or rude.

TOP TIP

Beware: the messages that we provide through body language may be very different to what we are saying.

Positive body language

Non-verbal communication is commonly referred to as body language.When speaking to clients, always maintain good eye contact; this shows that you are paying attention and are interested in them. Always smile while you are speaking. This puts the client at ease and makes them feel welcome. This can be particularly helpful and comforting to them as they may be feeling shy or unsure of themselves. It may even be their first visit to the salon and everything may be feeling very new or alien to them.

We express ourselves with body language through posture and gestures. Here are some of the most common:

◆ Slouching looks unprofessional.

◆ Folded or crossed arms can display a closed mind or defensiveness.

◆ Scratching behind the ear or the back of the neck indicates uncertainty.

◆ Inspecting the fingernails or looking at your watch is rude and indicates boredom or vanity.

◆ Talking with your hand in front your mouth may make the listener think you lack confidence.

◆ Shifting from foot to foot may indicate that you feel guilty about something.

TOP TIP

Time always passes more quickly for a client when there is something to read or look at. Always make a point of offering the client something to read while they are waiting.

ACTIVITY

What is the client saying?

Gestures and posturing are not the only ways that we show how we are feeling. Facial expressions can show a lot too. Copy the table and complete the missing information to indicate what each facial expression means. Then answer the questions.

Facial expression	What does it mean or show?
Smiling	
Frowning	
Laughing	
Narrowing of the eyes	
Red cheeks and tight lips	

1   What kind of facial expressions would a client be making if they were confused?
2   What kind of facial expressions would a client be making if they were angry?

Supporting the clients

Show that you care by demonstrating your politeness and courtesy. Find out if the clients need anything. Always make a point of asking if they would like a drink or something to read whilst they are waiting. This shows that you have not forgotten them, even if their usual stylist is running a little late. Your courtesy and concern shows that you care.

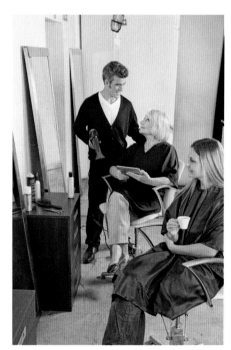

Bringing magazines and drinks is a simple task that puts the client at ease

Building professional relationships (Continued...)

Avoid confusing the clients

Always treat clients as individuals – different clients have differing needs. Always show patience – some clients may be elderly or hard of hearing and you may need to write things down for them or speak slowly. Never assume that everyone has the same understanding as you in your work. You may use special words or industry **jargon** with other colleagues, but will the client understand what a steamer is, or a graduated layer cut?

Treat clients' belongings with respect

The receptionist's job is to manage the reception area, to attend to calls and receive the clients. It is a busy area and there is always something going on. Your job role extends to assisting them in what they are doing and you can show this by helping with clients.

When clients arrive at the salon, they will usually be carrying bags or be wearing a coat or jacket. If these items are not kept tidy and put away safely, they could become a hazard to other people or get damaged or lost.

For safety and security reasons, when a client arrives at the reception, take their belongings and put them away safely. Remember, bags or shopping should not be stored on pegs or on shelves as they might fall on someone or damage the contents.

Coats and jackets should be hung up on pegs or coat hangers to prevent them from losing their tailoring and becoming misshapen.

Don't wait to be asked

If a client needs help or advice you should respond promptly and attend to their needs. Sometimes it will be something that you can do easily, such as turning the heat down on a dryer, or replacing a damp towel from around their shoulders with a clean, dry one, or bringing the client a selection of magazines or something to drink.

Sometimes you need to ask someone else If you don't know the answer to a question, ask someone who does – this is one of the most important salon rules. It is not a failing or weakness to ask others how things work, or what you need to do. On the contrary, it is a personal strength as it shows that you really take an interest in your work and want to get things right.

> **TOP TIP**
>
> Remember to hang clients' coats or jackets away from the salon's styling gowns as these could easily be damp or stained.

> **TOP TIP**
>
> Coats or jackets left draped over the back of the chair could easily get stained or damaged by chemicals used for hair services. If this were to occur, the client could make a claim for damages against the salon; this would be damaging to the salon's reputation.

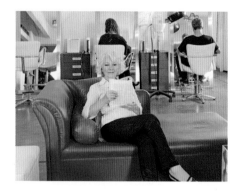

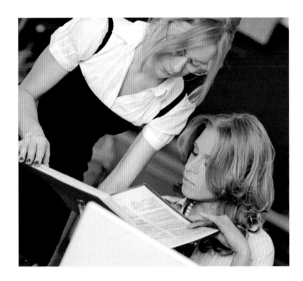

TOP TIP

Shopping bags crowded around the styling section or chairs are a slip and trip hazard. They also prevent the stylist from standing close enough to work on the clients hair.

Show willingness to help   Show that you are willing to provide a good service and gain the clients' trust in your abilities. Make sure that you always ask clients if they are comfortable and if they need anything. A good service will never go unnoticed. Whether it is the client, the other staff or your supervisor, people notice when others are making an effort – and when clients notice, they are more likely to express their gratitude and leave you a tip.

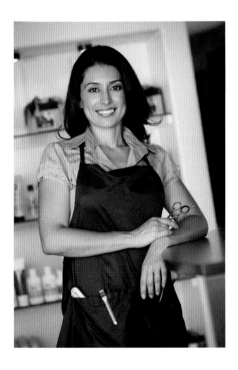

Building professional relationships (Continued...)

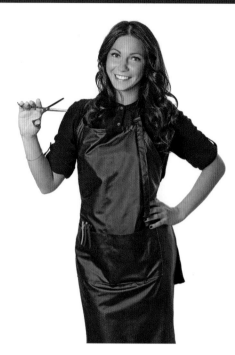

Look professional

An important aspect of professional communication is your appearance. What you wear and how you look can either reinforce the impression that you create with the client or destroy it altogether. This is why different jobs have different dress codes. Your salon will have its own dress code and expected standards of behaviour and appearance and you must abide by these rules. These will be the minimum levels that management will accept.

ACTIVITY

Copy the table and fill in the missing information to explore how different people in different jobs dress, and the reasons why.

Type of job	Dress code	Reason
a personal trainer in a fitness club		
a soldier on parade		
a chef cooking in a kitchen		
a beauty therapist		
a hairstylist or barber		
a checkout operator in a supermarket		

TOP TIP

Remember: You do not get a second chance to make a good first impression, so make it count!

ACTIVITY

Find out what is expected of you:

- what you should wear for work
- how you should look, in respect of your hair, make-up and general appearance
- how you should behave when working
- how you should respond to the clients.

Personal conduct

The salon or barber's shop is a professional environment and you are on show. The way in which you react to others and the respect that you show will be apparent not only by what you say, but how you say it. Treat others with a mutual professional respect, regardless of what you think or would like to say. Always conduct your work in a safe, professional manner; never fool around as this could put others at risk by your actions or negligence.

ACTIVITY

The table below lists a number of situations that could occur within the salon. Think about the things that could go wrong in each case. Copy the table and then:

◆ tick the first column if you can handle this yourself

◆ write down in the next column what you should do

◆ complete the third column if you cannot sort the problem and need to seek help.

Things that could go wrong	Can you sort this out yourself?	What should you do?	Who do you need to tell?
A client tells you that the colour on her head is beginning to feel sore.			
A client spills her coffee on the styling section shelf.			
You see that a client's towel is wet and has fallen to the floor.			
After a client's service has been finished, you find that they have left their purse behind.			
A client has had a perm and is waiting for it to develop, but you notice that the lotion is dripping down around their face.			
A stylist finishes a dry cut on a client and leaves the styling section untidy.			

Personal appearance is covered elsewhere in this book. See Chapter 3 Health and Safety, Dressing and behaving professionally, for more information.

BEST PRACTICE

◆ Do not rush or run around the salon.
◆ Always follow the manufacturer's instructions.
◆ Prepare and clean salon equipment before the clients arrive.
◆ Always use equipment for the purposes they were intended.
◆ Help prepare equipment or work areas for others.
◆ Keep the backwash area and basins clean and uncluttered.
◆ Replenish stock before it runs out.
◆ Behave professionally and sensibly.
◆ Do not endanger others in their work.
◆ Be responsible – spot hazards and take appropriate action to avoid injury to others.
◆ Remember that the client deserves respect, politeness and courtesy at all times.

TOP TIP

If in doubt always ask another member of staff. There will be many things that you do not know, but training is all about finding out and learning the things that you need to know in order to do your job correctly.

Being part of the team

All the staff in the salon work as a team, and your contributions are equally important. Without this joint effort, nothing will happen: the stylists, colourists and technicians will not be able to do their jobs and your fellow juniors will not be able to do theirs. Therefore, it is essential that you are friendly, helpful and respectful to other staff at all times. You may have your differences away from the salon floor, but you are now in a professional working environment and any animosity (bad feelings) must be left behind.

The friendships that you make out of work are different and made out of choice, whereas those acquaintances made through work are based on team associations. The two relationships are very different and require margins for tolerance, patience and acceptance, which happen to be part of your professional development within the job role.

Ask politely when you need help

The work carried out by staff within the salon depends on good communication, and that means politely asking others for help as well as offering help. Communication is a two-way process and it is always welcomed and returned. You ask for help or advice in a friendly manner and someone else responds to your needs with respect.

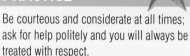

BEST PRACTICE

Be courteous and considerate at all times; ask for help politely and you will always be treated with respect.

Help willingly and promptly when asked

Good team working promotes a happy salon, and in turn, this creates an atmosphere that everyone will sense. On the other hand, a team that does not work together in harmony creates a stilted or strained bad atmosphere that clients will notice. You can help to prevent this from happening by always being willing to provide your assistance. Your eagerness and promptness to take part or help will not go unnoticed and will pay you back in the longer term.

TOP TIP

Always make good use of your time when you are in the salon. Sometimes you will have to juggle what you are doing as you may be asked to do one job while carrying out another for someone else:

◆ Keep a list of the different tasks you have been asked to do and that way you won't get into trouble for forgetting anything.

◆ Find out what jobs have priority – some things are more important or urgent. Do these things first.

◆ If you do not understand your task, ask someone to explain it right away.

◆ If you have to leave something halfway through, make sure that you complete it at the earliest convenient moment.

Only do jobs that you have been trained to do

Safety is always your employer's first consideration and many things will have gone on behind the scenes to make the place that you work in fit for purpose. However, that does not mean that work is always hazard free. Providing a public access to premises for a place of work always creates situations where accidents or hazards can occur, so you play an important role in helping to prevent those hazards from occurring. One way in which you can do this is to only do the jobs that you have been trained to do.

Tell your supervisor about any problems

Whenever you do encounter something new, or are unsure about doing something, tell either your supervisor or a senior member of staff, or ask for their assistance.

ACTIVITY

Match each statement on the left with its corresponding statement on the right and write down the correct sentences.

A	Relationships at work are based upon		1	personal preferences and choice
B	Friendships outside work are based upon		2	effective communication takes place
C	Customer care is built on		3	mutual respect and teamwork
D	Good customer relations occur when		4	professionalism and personal service
E	Teamwork takes place when		5	all the staff do their jobs efficiently

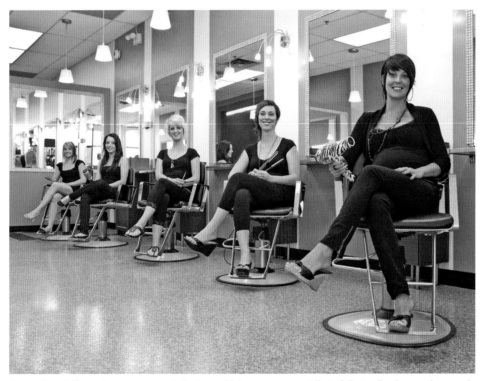

As a salon staff member you are part of a team. Make sure you contribute fully to all salon services, and are willing and friendly. You will learn a great deal about your profession and enjoy the teamwork.

Developing yourself within the job role

Know your own abilities and limitations

Being able to self-assess your own skills at work is an important part of your ongoing development and meeting your training targets. The key to doing your job and performing your team role properly is knowing what you do well and what you do not. On the surface, some tasks seem very simple and others seem very hard.

Why is that? Tasks that we do repeatedly become simpler. However, jobs that we do less often or dislike are the ones where we feel out of our comfort zone, and that uncertainty or self-doubt makes us feel that we cannot do them properly. Assessing your own strengths and weaknesses requires you to be realistic and honest with yourself about your capabilities. You need to define those jobs that you know and do well and those that you do not. The list of things that you do not do well forms the basis for creating targets for your **personal development plan**.

How well are you doing?

You can find out how well you are getting on through feedback from your work colleagues. As you work with them on a day-to-day basis, they will be able to tell you how well you are doing. However, as they are also friends, their comments will probably only cover the positives as they won't want to hurt your feelings. Ultimately, your work supervisor will be the one who has a very clear idea of what you can do, where you are now and where you need to be. At work, this assessment of your skills is called **appraisal**.

TOP TIP

For more information about National Vocational Qualifications for hairdressing, see www.habia.org

Learning new things

At work you have to learn everything that is related to the job. Some of these things are fun and easy to learn, but others may be more difficult to follow or understand, or just plain boring! You will find that learning opportunities present themselves in all sorts of ways and you should make the most of these in order to get on well. Learning opportunities fall into two categories: the ones that rely upon your participation in organized training events and others that rely upon your ability to learn through informal, day-to-day routine activities.

Formal, organized learning and training could take place during normal work hours, or arranged as an evening or outside-of-work event. Most salons have specific times for staff training, usually model evenings, role-plays or demonstrations and presentations. For example, a junior stylist may demonstrate how a professional shampoo is carried out for you to practise afterwards. Alternatively, a manufacturer's field technician may do an in-salon product demonstration.

You will find that you learn most things informally through your everyday duties; you will be seeing how other staff do things, how staff communicate with clients and handle situations. You will hear how they offer services, recommend products and provide advice.

ACTIVITY

What can you learn here?

The table below lists a number of situations that give you opportunities to learn. Copy the table. Think about what is happening in each situation and then complete the missing information. When you have finished, check your answers with your work supervisor.

Opportunities to learn new things	What can you learn from this?	What questions would you ask?
Watching a junior carrying out a shampoo		
Helping the receptionist		
Helping the stylist by passing up		
Watching the stylist mixing chemicals		
Listening to a stylist conduct a consultation		
Helping the junior refill the shampoos and conditioners		

ACTIVITY

Find out your salon's policy for communicating with other staff and clients in your salon. Write the answer in your portfolio.

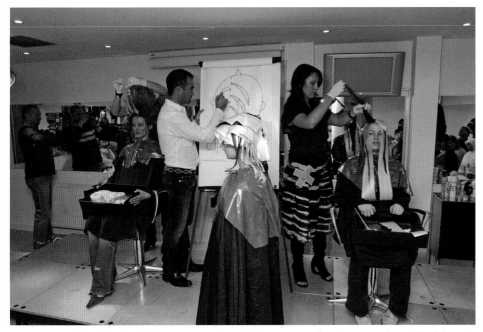

Learning through a formal training event at a salon will give you great hands-on experience. Don't forget to add such training sessions to your personal development plan.

Developing yourself within the job role (Continued...)

Reviewing your progress

Earlier in this chapter we used the term appraisal. The appraisal interview is not an inquisition or a way of having a go at you. It is a positive and professional process and your contribution is important. The appraisal process is a way of looking at an individual's abilities, assessing their needs and mutually agreeing a course of action.

Appraisal

A business needs to do well in order to survive and you are an essential part of that team. You will not know how you are doing unless someone in a supervisory role gives you feedback. The appraisal process provides this mechanism.

In order for the business to do well and keep everyone employed, it must create a profit. If a business does not make a profit then it soon ceases to exist! Therefore, the business must achieve its performance targets in order to survive and prevail. You are part of that entity and you must achieve your personal targets so that the business can achieve its own targets. Your personal targets and objectives are set out within your appraisal, which will:

- review the progress that has been made since the last appraisal

- check your current personal performance

- agree and set new targets for the next period, moving on from what has already been learned.

Your review of progress will be done with your supervisor during your appraisal. This will give you the opportunity to see where you are now and where you need to be.

Where you are now   When you started work you received a job description. This is a sort of checklist of the things that you should be doing or working towards. Now, depending how long you have been in the role, you may be able to say that you have covered many of the duties already. Some of these things will be done well and others perhaps not so well. Your appraisal will be an opportunity to review these things and discuss your progress and competence in each of the tasks associated with them. You can then discuss the things that you need to work on and do in the future. Be positive and willing to contribute; discuss the things that you feel you do well and have completed. Be objective and not defensive as this is an aid to your personal development and not a personal attack.

Job description: Junior/Trainee

Location   Cutz 'n Curlz

Main purpose of job: to provide good customer care at all times, maintain a good standard of client care and follow salon's standard training practices and procedures

The job holder should:

> have a professional level of interpersonal/communication skills
>
> be a willing and conscientious team member
>
> be willing to participate in personal development activities during work hours and on training evenings
>
> achieve designated performance targets
>
> undertake duties requested by senior staff

The job holder should maintain company policy in respect of:

> personal standards of health/hygiene
>
> personal standards of appearance/conduct
>
> operating safely while at work
>
> timekeeping and service provision
>
> company image and public promotion
>
> company security practices and procedures

Sample job description

Where you need to be   After the 'where you are now' has been covered, it is time to think towards the future. The rest of the appraisal will look at things that you need to be doing up to the next appraisal date. You will be talking about new targets and ways that you could go about achieving them. The targets could cover a wide range of things. Some targets could relate to retail sales or in-salon promotions, while others could be training targets. For example, be able to use flat brushes for blow-drying, or be able to put hair into rope plaits.

Developing yourself within the job role (Continued...)

ACTIVITY

Strengths and weaknesses

Being able to self-assess your own strengths and weaknesses is fundamental to moving forwards. If you do not know what you are good at, how do you know what to improve? This activity will help you to do this. Copy and complete the table by putting a tick in the appropriate boxes for each of the skills listed. When you have filled in the information, ask your work supervisor to check your responses.

Personal Skill	I do this	I do this well	I don't do this	I don't do this very well
Communicating with clients				
Communicating with work colleagues				
Helping other staff in their work				
Doing things myself without having to be told all the time				
Dealing with clients and handling their queries				
Tidying the salon and keeping things clean				

TOP TIP

Your salon has a procedure for appeals and grievances. See the company's handbook or speak to your work supervisor or employer for more information.

Your salon's appeal and grievance procedure

A grievance is a complaint or objection to something that has happened. It could occur for a number of reasons where you may feel that you have been treated unfairly, or wronged in some way, and in a work situation this could relate to many things. If you have a grievance at work, you must deal with the situation professionally. Be calm and sensible and take it up with your work supervisor first. If that would be a problem for you, seek independent advice on how to deal with the situation.

Your salon will have its own way of implementing grievance or disciplinary procedures, and you should receive this information during your induction. The procedure will cover the following issues:

◆ conflict at work between staff

◆ unfair (or presumed unfair) treatment at work (e.g. being asked to do tasks beyond your abilities or unsafe practices)

◆ discrimination in any situation.

SUMMARY

Now you have finished this chapter you should have a clearer picture of everything relating to team working and working together. In particular, you should now have a basic understanding of:

✓ communicating professionally with clients and colleagues

✓ the ways in which you can work to promote team building and harmony

✓ the ways in which you can work to minimize conflict with other staff

✓ how you can develop yourself within the job role.

In addition, you will understand how these principles will enable you to provide satisfactory and enjoyable services to all the salon's clients.

REVISION QUESTIONS

Q1. Copy and complete this sentence: The correct name for a salon or barber shop customer is a _____ .

Fill in the blank

Q2. Relationships at work are different to those outside of work?

True or False

Q3. Which of the following are examples of good teamwork?
(You may choose more than one answer.)

asking for help politely from others ☐ a

preparing trolleys with curlers ☐ b

sitting at the reception desk ☐ c

finding ways to avoid jobs ☐ d

finding ways to learn new things ☐ e

cleaning the brushes for the stylists ☐ f

Q4. Goodwill is shown by treating clients in a kind, friendly way?

True or False

Q5. Which of the following would *not* be a feature of a self-development plan?
(You may choose more than one answer.)

self-improvement ○ a

setting targets ○ b

personal objectives ○ c

grievance procedures ○ d

5 Reception

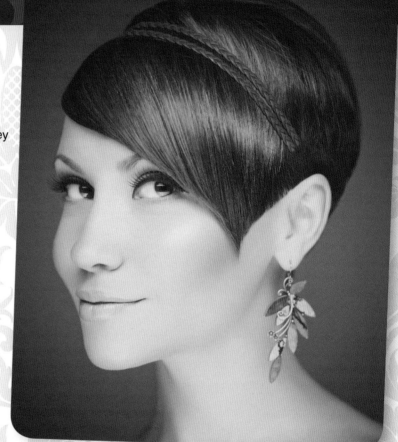

LEARNING OBJECTIVES

When you have finished this chapter you should:

◆ be able to make clients feel welcome when they arrive

◆ be able to carry out salon reception duties

◆ know the salon's services, products and their prices

◆ be able to make appointments accurately

◆ be able to communicate professionally.

KEY TERMS

appointment system

body language

client care

confidentiality

Data Protection Act 1998

effective communication

goodwill

INFORMATION COVERED IN THIS CHAPTER

PRACTICAL SKILLS

Learn how to make appointments for clients face-to-face or on the telephone.

Find out what clients want by asking the right questions.

Learn how to monitor stationery stocks and report/replace items before they run out.

Learn how to take bills and record sales.

Learn how to calculate bills and give accurate change.

Make sure that you update the clients' records.

UNDERPINNING KNOWLEDGE

Know your salon's ranges of products and services.

Understand the features of positive body language.

Know how to communicate effectively and professionally.

Understand the salon's appointment system and the ways of making appointments.

Know the salon's procedures for handling payments from clients.

Know how to maintain confidentiality when handling client information.

INTRODUCTION

The receptionist is the first and last person to see a client. If you are working in reception or assisting the receptionist you will be on show. Therefore, the way you act and communicate has a direct effect on the clients and how they are made to feel.

The receptionist has an important role to play, and if you are helping them you will be taking messages, making and recording appointments and providing clients with information, or making them drinks while they are waiting. Your role will be equally important as you are on show too; you are the face of the salon to arriving clients and support for those people making enquiries on the telephone. This is your chance to make a positive and professional impression.

Looking after the reception area

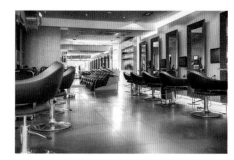

First impressions

The reception area is the first point of contact that the clients have with the salon and you may be the first person in the salon that they meet. Their first impression will be based on what they see and the way they are handled, how you greet them and your general approach.

Keeping all areas clean and tidy
You will have to show that you can keep the reception area neat and tidy, greet people entering the salon, deal with their questions and make straightforward appointments. You will be using your communication skills when people come into the salon, or when speaking to them on the telephone. This is a very important part of the business and you will be contributing to the overall team effort.

Salon tidiness is essential and maintenance in reception is equally important: a clean, attractive reception and retail display conveys a message of professionalism and pride. Add to this a warm smile, a friendly 'Hello, how can I help you?' and good eye contact, and instant, good customer care takes place.

It is your duty to make sure that the reception area is clean and tidy at all times. Make sure that carpets are vacuumed before the salon gets busy and that tiled areas are swept or mopped (and kept dry) throughout the day. Keep the displays fully stocked and the shelves free of dust. Check retail products for condition and ensure price labels are clearly visible. Attractive retail products will encourage clients to look at what is on offer and find out more.

The **appointment system** is in continual use, so stationery, pens and messages can be left around on the reception desk. The desk is the focal point of any reception and its level of organization will affect how clients view the salon.

Personal appearance
The effort we put into getting ready for work reflects the pride we take in our jobs. Sometimes we have to wear clothes that would not be our personal choice, but professional standards and salon image come first. Dress neatly in your salon's uniform or according to the dress code and make sure your hair is clean and well-groomed at all times.

TOP TIP
Put yourself in the client's position. What do they see? Are the product labels facing the front? Is supporting product information available? Is everything clean? How would you feel if you picked up a product and it left a dirty, dusty ring on the shelf?

See Chapter 3 for more information on health, safety and hygiene.

BEST PRACTICE

Checklist for salon tidiness:

- desk dusted and tidied before clients arrive
- appointment diary close to hand and ready for use
- card payment receipt rolls and till rolls replenished and spares available
- stationery stocks checked and replenished
- shelves and retail products dusted or wiped
- missing items or low stock levels replaced or reported
- damaged or faulty product packaging removed and reported to the manager
- products rearranged and gaps in product lines removed from displays
- product information and pricing is up to date, close at hand and easy to read
- product promotions are clearly displayed, public information is available and the correct product items are arranged appropriately according to the current offer or promotion.

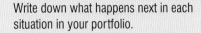

ACTIVITY

Client communication

1   Watch how the people in the reception area deal with clients and enquiries. What do you notice about the way they deal with the following situations?

   ◆ A client arrives at reception.
   ◆ The telephone rings.
   ◆ Someone leaves a message for one of the stylists.
   ◆ A client is browsing the products on the retail display.

Write down what happens next in each situation in your portfolio.

2   What are you expected to do in respect to:

   a   maintaining the reception area
   b   attending to people and enquiries
   c   making appointments?

> **TOP TIP**
>
> Dust the products on the retail displays regularly: no one wants to handle products that look murky and dull, regardless of how fabulous they are and what they can do.

Monitoring stationery and product levels

The reception area is always busy with clients arriving or wanting to pay their bill; the telephone is often ringing with clients wanting to make appointments. Therefore the desk must be well organized. Stationery, such as memo pads, pens and till rolls or electronic payment machine stationery, needs checking every morning before the salon opens and restocking throughout the day.

Don't forget the product information: promotional information helps to sell retail products. It provides clients with relevant information in professionally produced leaflets, booklets and brochures. Make sure that all current promotions have their supporting information at hand. In busy, thriving salons, the contents of the retail displays are going to change throughout the day. The salon may start out with fully stocked displays, but as the items are sold, gaps will start appearing and product lines may run out. A well-stocked display is more appealing than one with gaps. If you notice any shortages, get some replacements from the stock storage room.

ACTIVITY

Positive and negative impressions

Put yourself in the client's position and think about the following statements. What things would give you a positive impression and what things would give you a negative impression of the business? Copy the statements into your portfolio and give an example of a positive and negative impression for each one.

   ◆ You open the door and walk into reception.
   ◆ You walk over to look at the products.
   ◆ A member of staff makes eye contact with you.
   ◆ You want to make an appointment.
   ◆ You feel confused about what you are hearing.
   ◆ You ask to speak to the manager.

Looking after the reception area (Continued...)

Looking out for faulty or damaged products

Sometimes accidents happen and product packaging can be damaged. If you find any products that are faulty or damaged, report them to the person in charge of the stock and then clear up any spillages or leaks.

Look for faulty stock as you prepare it for display. Look out for leaking products in the delivery packaging. If any contents are missing, a product cannot be sold. Retail products are often packed in sealed boxes in multiples of 6s, 10s or 12s, and each one has a cost to the salon. All damaged items can be returned to the supplier and the costs reimbursed, so by reporting them to your supervisor, you will be showing your efficiency and making savings for the salon.

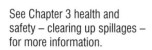

See Chapter 3 health and safety – clearing up spillages – for more information.

ACTIVITY

Retail products in your place of work

Copy and complete the following table for some of the retail products in your salon.

Retail product name	Who makes the product?	What is it used for?	How much does it cost?

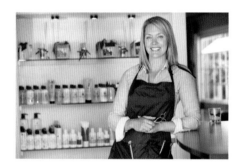

Demonstrating good customer care

Some salons offer drinks as part of their service policy. Make sure that you offer the client whatever your salon includes as part of its customer service policy. Always make a point of asking if they would like something to read.

A stylebook is particularly helpful, as it may save valuable time when the stylist does the client's consultation, or it might even get them thinking about something new. If they do not want to look at styles, perhaps get them a magazine instead.

TOP TIP

Show clients you care about them by offering a drink while they are waiting. It shows that they have been noticed and not forgotten. Remember to ask how they take it.

ACTIVITY

Find out what the general standards of hospitality are in your salon or shop.

◆ What is the customer service policy at your salon?

◆ What aspects of the service are complimentary?

Write your answers in your portfolio.

ACTIVITY

The reception area is the hub of the salon: clients arrive, calls are received, visitors arrive, bills are paid and appointments are made. Match these tasks to their operations by writing out the correct sentences.

A	Retail products should be dusted daily…	1	…because handling information correctly is so important
B	Hairstyle books and magazines are useful…	2	…because people don't buy or handle dirty items
C	Offer clients a drink or magazines…	3	…because we must convey a professional image and service
D	Appointments books are essential…	4	…because they help people describe a new look
E	Good communication is essential…	5	…because sometimes they have to wait for a while
F	Messages should always be passed on to the right person…	6	…because they organize the stylist's day

TOP TIP

When you find magazines for the client, pick the latest, rather than just picking up the first one you see.

Effective communication

Effective communication is essential in a service industry and it is crucial to the businesses success at reception. The way that you address people who arrive at the salon is going to leave them with a lasting impression. Your communication needs to be clear and effective. Some people are not as able as others, so sometimes you will have to speak a little more slowly or perhaps a little louder. In any situation, make sure that you have been understood by confirming the details back to them.

Communication is about passing on information. The information in a message can provide details, advice or answers. Be polite and positive at all times; your ability to do your job will be assumed (rightly or wrongly) by the way in which you communicate with the clients. When you speak:

◆ in a strained voice: this indicates that 'I'm under pressure here, don't bother me now'

◆ in a raised voice: this indicates that 'I'm angry about something that has just happened'

◆ in a friendly voice: this indicates that 'I'm helpful, professional and I'm ready to serve'.

Not everyone who arrives at the salon is a client, and unless you establish this first, you could embarrass yourself. You need to find out with whom you are dealing and what they want. The simplest greeting for a face-to-face communication is to smile and say, 'How may I help you?' This polite and friendly greeting provides a catch-all phrase for any visitor and allows them to respond: 'I have an appointment to see…' or 'I would like to make an appointment…' or 'Is Jill busy? I would like a quick word.' Then, depending on their response, you can adapt your reply.

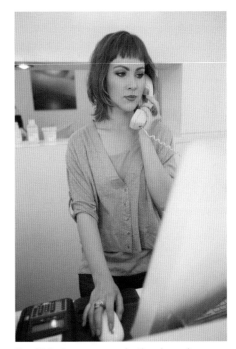

Good telephone communication depends on your voice, tone and delivery

Attending to clients and enquiries

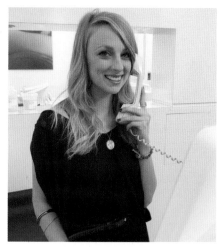

You are the salon's representative when speaking on the telephone

When a client arrives for their appointment, make sure that you attend to them promptly. Confirm their appointment and the time and then direct them to a seat. Always make a point of making them feel welcome. People dislike waiting for anything, and this can start their experience off on the wrong foot. If you think of those times when you have to wait in a queue, or wait to be seen by the doctor, those feelings and memories will spring to mind.

One of the greatest gifts that you can give anyone is your time. You can demonstrate this by being aware of other people's time, so when a client arrives for an appointment you must inform the stylist immediately. If a client has to wait because a stylist is running late, you can at least inform them so that they can look at their alternatives.

ACTIVITY

Write your answers to the following questions in your portfolio:

1   **a.** In what situation would you need to speak more slowly to a client?
    b. What signs would the client be showing that required you to do this?
2   **a.** When would you need to speak more loudly to a client?
    b. What signs would the client be showing that required you to do this?
3   **a.** What signs would a client be showing if they were confused?
    b. What signs might they be showing if they were angry?

TOP TIP

Always keep a message pad close to the telephone: writing messages on the appointment book is unprofessional and must be avoided at all costs.

Referring enquiries you can't handle

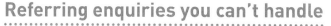

Enquiries made either in person 'face-to-face', or on the telephone should be handled in the same way. In both instances you need to respond promptly and politely. If you do not know the answer to a question, ask someone who does – accurate information is essential. So stop and listen to what the customer says. Hear the request and act on the information or instruction. A simple misunderstanding could result in giving or recording the wrong information and might turn into a disaster. Imagine if the client turns up on the wrong day and cannot be done because her stylist is too busy!

It is even more difficult on the telephone because callers can only gain an impression of the salon from the person they speak to on the telephone. This person becomes the salon's sole representative, acting on behalf of the business, and their ability to listen, speak clearly, respond to requests and act upon information is critical to the salon's **goodwill** and image.

Smile when you answer the telephone – people will 'hear' the friendliness in your voice. Speak clearly so that the caller understands everything you say. After listening to the caller's request, confirm the main points back to the caller. This summarizes the information and ensures that all details are correct. Keep the call short: calls cost money and waste valuable salon time.

There will be occasions when you need to seek assistance or advice from others. Recognizing situations when you are unable to help is not a failure – it is all part of professional communication. An example might be when stock arrives and a signature is required for taking delivery and accepting the condition of the goods.

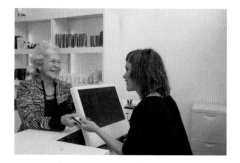

Taking messages for others

You will sometimes need to take a message on behalf of someone else. It is essential that these messages are accurate and delivered promptly to the appropriate person. When taking messages, always make sure that you record as much detail as you can in relation to the message:

◆ who the message is for

◆ the date and time received

◆ who has taken it

◆ the purpose or content of the message.

Handling information in a confidential way

Certain circumstances and situations need special care and attention, and probably the most important aspect of professional communication is **confidentiality**. During your day-to-day work, it is possible that you will come into contact with information that others consider private. It is important that you recognize these situations and handle them accordingly. This confidential information will occur in numerous ways: during routine conversations between staff or clients, and from business contacts and inquirers. Whatever the source, you must not pass on personal or potentially sensitive information to anyone.

Confidential information includes:

◆ the details within clients' records

◆ clients' and staff's personal details such as name, address and telephone number

◆ financial information relating to the business.

A client's confidential information is protected by law and the **Data Protection Act 1998** allows the salon to obtain, hold and use personal data, providing that the information is kept secure. The Act upholds the client's rights by preventing the unlawful disclosure of information to another person or business entity.

TOP TIP

A personal conversation is also confidential and definitely private. People tend to talk about all sorts of things when they are in the salon and anything that you overhear must remain private.

See Appendix 1 for more information on the Data Protection Act 1998.

ACTIVITY

What is your salon or shop's policy and procedures for:

a   maintaining confidentiality

b   taking messages

c   making and recording appointments

d   client care at reception.

What might happen if you broke confidentiality?

Write your answers in your portfolio.

TOP TIP

Personal information is private information. Never spread gossip or talk about other people's personal conversations. It is strictly confidential.

Making appointments

It is essential that appointments are made accurately and promptly every time, regardless of whether they are made by telephone or face-to-face. Before you can schedule appointments, you must have an idea of the services available. Each salon or barber's shop offers a unique 'menu' of services. Different stylists or barbers will have different abilities and skills, and so might be available only for certain services at certain levels. Get to know the variety of services, the timings and costs that the salon or shop and its stylists or barbers have to offer.

BEST PRACTICE

When you make appointments for clients, try to offer a range of dates at different times. If a client cannot make a weekday appointment at 3:30pm she may be at work, so offering another day at the same time will probably be unsuitable too.

ACTIVITY

This activity is linked with the appointment system. It relates to the services and their costs at your place of work. Copy the table into your portfolio and fill in the details for your salon.

Service	Service abbreviation	Which stylists or barbers do this?	How long does it take?	How much does it cost?
dry cut				
wet cut				
blow-dry (short hair)				
blow-dry (long hair)				
shampoo and set				
T–section highlights				
full head highlights				
roots colour				
full head colour				
permanent wave				

BEST PRACTICE

Always introduce yourself when handling calls. People like to speak to someone they can associate with, not strangers or machines!

Dealing with requests promptly and politely

Making appointments need not be difficult. It is about matching client requests with the time available. You want to help the customer to make the booking, while bearing in mind the time it will take and who will be providing the service.

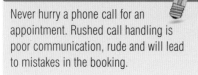

TOP TIP

Never hurry a phone call for an appointment. Rushed call handling is poor communication, rude and will lead to mistakes in the booking.

Telephone calls   You should always remember to smile, as people can hear the friendliness in your voice. Now say something like: 'Good morning/afternoon, Head Masters hair salon. This is Hayley speaking, how can I help you?' A friendly but positive approach will immediately give a professional image of both the salon and yourself. Ideally, you should let the telephone ring two or three times before answering; this allows the caller, who may be new to the salon or who may be an older person, the time to prepare what they want to say.

Visits in person   The most popular way for clients to contact the salon is by telephone, but clients will often call in to the salon in person to make an appointment. You need to be ready for the 'drop in' spontaneous client. When someone walks into the reception area, they might be feeling a little uncomfortable or uneasy. You can dispel these feelings of uncertainty by making eye contact, smiling and attending to them promptly and politely. The common greeting of: 'Good morning/afternoon. How can I help you?' will do one of the following:

◆ confirm that they have a booked appointment

◆ show that they have not got an appointment but would like to make one

◆ let you know that they are not a client but have other reasons for calling.

Accurately recording appointments

Each salon has its own system for making appointments but, generally speaking, appointment scheduling is completed in such a way as to maximize the time available with appropriate staff members. Bearing this in mind, you should always remain ready, prompt and polite in attending to the client's requests. When you have found out what the caller wants, you are ready to make the appointment by asking the following questions:

◆ 'On what day would you like the appointment?'

◆ 'What time do you have in mind?'

◆ 'What would you like to have done?'

◆ 'Which stylist is that with/would you like to see?'

Each time you ask one of the questions above, you are narrowing the possible responses; you are leading the conversation in a controlled professional way and reducing the chances of making a mistake. The four questions above very quickly allow you to get to the:

◆ right day in the appointment system

◆ available times for services

◆ type of service required by the client

◆ availability of their stylist to do the job.

Now you have to work out if there is enough time to make the appointment for the client. This is often the most difficult part of making appointments, because some require a single block of time, whereas others take multiple blocks.

For example, a booking for a haircut or a blow-dry is a single block appointment. A colour or perm appointment is more complex because these can straddle other appointments to allow for the colour or perm to develop, allowing the stylist to do something else in between.

Date: Friday 12th September

Time	Clare
9.00	
9.15	
9.30	Taylor BD
9.45	
10.00	
10.15	
10.30	

In this example we see a single block appointment made by a regular client on **Friday 13th September** at **9.30** with **Clare** for **Mrs. Taylor** for a **blow dry**

Date: Friday 12th September

Time	Clare
9.00	Summers HLT
9.15	0123 456789
9.30	Taylor BD
9.45	
10.00	Summers CBD
10.15	
10.30	

Here we see an additional appointment with contact details made on **Friday 13th September** at **9.00** with **Clare** for Miss **Summers** for a **highlights T-section**, which now straddles the Taylor appointment and is booked back with Clare to do a cut and blow dry at 10.00

ACTIVITY

Role-play making appointments with your colleagues. Ask your supervisor if you can use the salon's/shop's appointment system to make the test bookings. Working with a colleague, take it in turns to make appointments (in pencil) both for callers on the telephone and in person. Make a range of appointments covering a variety of services. When you have finished get your supervisor to check that you have completed the information correctly.

Making appointments (Continued...)

Appointment details

Make sure that when the booking is made you record the information accurately and clearly and that you have considered all the factors:

- date and time
- the client's name
- service required
- stylist required
- client contact details

Ask for help

When you are not sure, it is always better to ask someone else than to make an incorrect booking. Some appointments are straightforward, whereas others may involve some complex scheduling or assistance from the stylist involved. If you are in any doubt, ask the stylist. They will know by looking at the client's hair how long they will need to complete the work. Sometimes the client will need a consultation prior to the appointment, say for extensions or 'hair-up'. These types of appointments require the stylist to have particular materials to complete the work and they may not be in stock, so will need to be ordered.

Difficult or angry clients If you can see by a client's face (by their expressions) that they are not happy about something, it is not your job to try sort out their problem. Simply ask them to take a seat and then find a senior member of staff to deal with their concerns.

Confirming and recording details correctly

Record the client's name clearly in the appointment system alongside the requested service, and check that it is booked for the correct day and time with the appropriate stylist. As a matter of customer service, it is also useful to give the client an approximate idea of service cost and length of appointment time. At the end, summarize all the information back to the client, to check it is correct.

TOP TIP

Sure that there are pencils, pens and eraser or correction fluid at the desk. Alterations to appointments happen all the time and you need to make those changes right away: do not leave it until later or it might not get done.

TOP TIP

When clients arrive in person, look for a positive response (e.g. nodding) when you confirm the appointment details. This will show that they understand what you are saying.

BEST PRACTICE

If the client has come in to the salon or shop to make the appointment, give them an appointment card as a token of good service and as a prompt. This provides a physical copy of the appointment and another way of ensuring that all the facts are correct.

ACTIVITY

Self-assessment

Do not attempt this activity until you have had some experience of reception work. Copy the checklist below and use it to self-assess. Ask your supervisor to check your responses.

Task	I do this well	I do this OK	I can't do this yet	Supervisor's comment
answering the telephone				
dealing with enquiries				
making appointments				
keeping reception clean				
restocking retail products				
restocking stationery items				

SUMMARY

Now you have finished this chapter you should have a clearer picture of all the essential aspects associated with working and helping in reception. In particular, you should now have a basic understanding of:

✓ meeting and greeting the salon's clients

✓ making appointments for clients

✓ taking messages and handling calls and enquiries

✓ the payment systems that are available within salons.

In addition, you will understand how these processes will enable you to work more efficiently and effectively in face-to-face situations with customers.

REVISION QUESTIONS

Q1. Copy and complete this sentence: All customer information and data is _____ information.

Fill in the blank

Q2. The reception should be clean and attractive throughout the working day?

True or False

Q3. Which of the following are not reception duties? (You may choose more than one answer.)

cleaning the product displays ☐ a

replenishing the till rolls ☐ b

making appointments ☐ c

tidying the roller trolleys ☐ d

refilling the shampoos ☐ e

answering the telephone ☐ f

Q4. If stock is delivered to reception you should always try to move it?

True or False

Q5. Which of the following should be offered to a client who arrives a little late for their appointment? (Choose one answer.)

an alternative appointment time ◯ a

a seat and a drink whilst they are waiting ◯ b

an alternative service ◯ c

a complimentary product for home use ◯ d

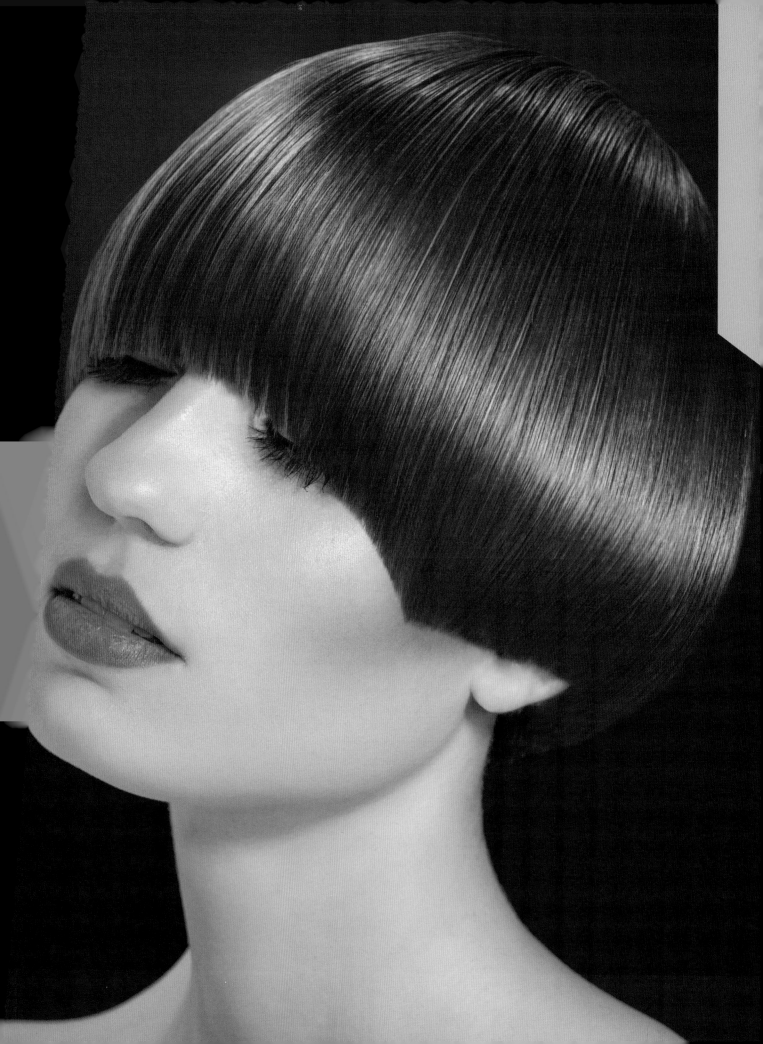

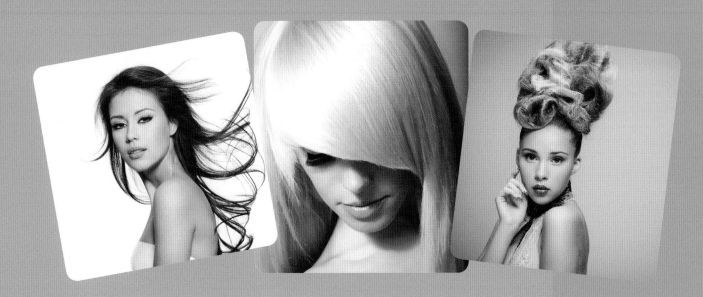

PART TWO

Practical skills

When your client arrives for their appointment they are warmly greeted by the salon receptionist. First impressions are vital, so it is important that their experience is a positive one from the moment they arrive until the moment they leave. After being checked in by the receptionist, you take over and play an active role in their care by performing or assisting with all the services that the client has requested.

When your client is sitting comfortably at the workstation, they need to be prepared for the services they have booked, and you must give them due care and attention. In the following chapters, you will be introduced to the skills and knowledge you need to master so that you can help the stylist do their job efficiently and effectively. Make sure you look and act professionally at all times, smile often, and remember: practice makes perfect!

6 Shampooing and Conditioning Hair

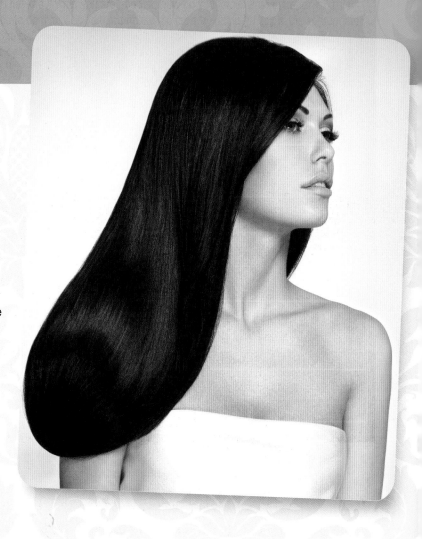

LEARNING OBJECTIVES

When you have finished this chapter you should:

◆ be able to work safely when shampooing and conditioning

◆ be able to prepare the client for the service

◆ be able to shampoo and condition hair

◆ know how and when to use different massage techniques

◆ know the salon's products for different hair types and conditions.

KEY TERMS

antioxidant conditioner

cortex

cuticle

dermatitis

detergent

effleurage

friction

hydrophilic

hydrophobic

penetrating conditioner

petrissage

pH balance

rotary

steamers

surface conditioner

surface tension

INFORMATION COVERED IN THIS CHAPTER

PRACTICAL SKILLS

Find out which products you need to use and get them ready.

Learn to work safely and efficiently while providing the service.

Learn how to shampoo different types and lengths of hair.

Learn how to condition different types and lengths of hair.

Learn how to behave professionally after consultation.

UNDERPINNING KNOWLEDGE

Know your salon's ranges of products for shampooing and conditioning.

Know how to prepare and protect the client correctly for shampooing and conditioning.

Understand the effects of shampooing and conditioning on the hair.

Know how to communicate with clients professionally.

INTRODUCTION

Almost every salon service involves shampooing and conditioning at some point, and in most situations it provides the starting point. Therefore, this service is both the first experience and first impression that the client will get of the salon, and your role in providing this service is vitally important in helping to make it a good one.

This chapter will explain the things that you need to know and do, so that you can be confident in getting it right for each client, every time you shampoo and condition hair.

What does shampooing and conditioning do to hair?

How do shampoos work?

All types of shampoo contain a common cleaning agent. They also contain other things, such as oils, moisturizers and flyaway control, but this varies depending on the hair type they are designed for.

The action of shampooing does three things:

◆ **Detergent** in the shampoo cleans the hair by removing dust, dirt and grease.

◆ Shampooing prepares the hair for further services.

◆ Warm water opens the **cuticle** of the hair so that conditioners are more effective.

Surface conditioner does three things:

◆ They smooth the cuticle layer, making it easier to detangle.

◆ They add moisture to hair, making it look healthy and giving it shine.

◆ They change the chemical properties of hair by restoring its natural pH.

Penetrating conditioner works deeper within the hair's **cortex** to do all of the above and:

◆ Repairs damage to the structure of the hair caused by excessive heat or chemical processes, such as colours and lightening.

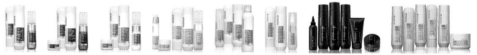

Shampoos come in a range of different formulations for different hair types and conditions

The cleaning component is a detergent with a long chemical name, usually abbreviated to SLS or TLS if you look at the ingredients list. However, the detergent within shampoo will not clean the hair on its own; it also needs water and some agitation, and that is where you come in. The water dampens the hair down and enables the shampoo to spread more easily, and you apply the agitation in the massage technique when you rub and scrub the dampened hair.

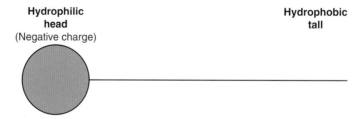

Hydrophilic head
(Negative charge)

Hydrophobic tall

A detergent molecule is like a polar magnet. One end has a negative (−) charge and is attracted to water (hydrophilic). The other end has a positive (+) charge and repels water (hydrophobic).

From this, you can see that three things are needed to make shampoo work:

◆ detergent – the cleaning component of shampoo

◆ water – to enable the shampoo to spread evenly over the hair

◆ rubbing action – within the massage techniques of **effleurage** and **rotary**.

The following images explain the physical/chemical properties of detergent molecules within shampoo and a short sequence of how they remove grease from a hair.

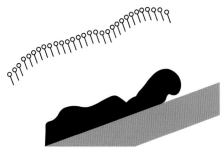

When molecules of detergent are spread through water, the hydrophobic (water fearing) ends are attracted to the grease.

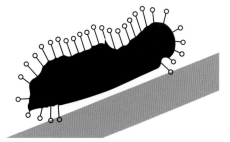

When the ends come into contact with the grease they stick all around its surface. The detergent breaks the **surface tension** of the grease and detaches it from the hair.

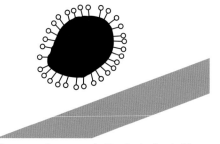

The grease is surrounded by the hydrophobic ends of the detergent and rolls up, lifting away from the hair and into the water.

> **TOP TIP**
>
> You can find out more information about dermatitis and health and safety legislation at www.hse.gov.uk

> **TOP TIP**
>
> Always follow the manufacturer's instructions when using any chemical products, and wear latex-free disposable gloves.

How do conditioners work?

Conditioners work in two ways:

◆ **Absorption** – relies on the condition of the hair. Dry hair is porous like a sponge; it has many tiny spaces within its internal structure. These areas *suck in* the conditioning elements, just as water is drawn into a sponge.

◆ **Attraction** – the hair has a minute electrical charge. During shampooing the detergent removes all traces of product, dirt and grease, leaving the surface of the hair in a positively charged state. This attracts the negative charge of conditioner, making it stick to the hair like a magnet.

This ionic attraction principle can be explained another way. Think of how balloons can be stuck to the wall by rubbing them vigorously on the sleeve of your jumper. This removes small electrical charges, now making the balloon stick to any surface!

> **TOP TIP**
>
> Always use a funnel to top up the shampoos and conditioners at the basin. This will prevent spillage and unnecessary waste. Pouring from a five-litre container into a narrow-necked one-litre container is very difficult.

Working safely and efficiently

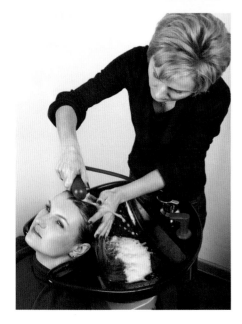

Protecting the client and their clothes

You must protect the client's clothes from spills and splashes with a clean, freshly laundered gown and towel. After taking the client's coat and bags and putting them away somewhere secure, you can put their gown on and place the towel around their shoulders, fixing it around the client's neck with a sectioning clip. Watch the towel in relation to the basin and the client's neck when shampooing. If there isn't enough towel between the basin and neck, water can seep down the client's neck and wet their clothes. Too much fabric will quickly become saturated, making the client uncomfortable and wetting their clothes.

The basin and seat must support the client's neck and back. It is very important that, after sitting the client at the basin, you check that they are comfortable. When the client is correctly seated, the basin should neither pinch or cause discomfort, nor should it allow water to leak over the rim.

Your posture

Your standing position is equally important from a safety point of view. You should stand close enough to the basin so that you can stand upright when:

See Chapter 3 Health and safety for more information on maintaining a high level of health, safety and hygiene throughout the shampooing and conditioning service.

◆ at a **side wash position**, where your arms and shoulders are positioned above your body and hips, without needing to twist or lean forwards

◆ at a **back wash position**, where your arms and shoulders are directly above your hips and feet and slightly behind the position of the client's head when they lie back.

You need to maintain the same posture throughout the shampoo or conditioning process, otherwise you will be exposing yourself to the risk of injury and longer term back condition or fatigue.

Keeping the basin area clean and safe to use

Remember to keep the work area clean and tidy at all times. All items should be removed from the sinks and side areas before any client sits at the basin. This includes removing:

HEALTH & SAFETY

Some injuries or neck complaints prevent the client from lying back at a basin. In some cases this has led to clients passing out when pressure is applied to the back of the neck. Before proceeding, ask your client if they know of any reason why they cannot use a backwards style wash-point.

◆ waste product containers, such as conditioners or shampoos

◆ colouring bowls, brushes and colouring products

◆ perming solutions or neutralizer in bottles or bowls, used end papers and sponges

◆ used neck wool, plastic caps and capes

◆ loose hair caught in the hair traps in the drain.

Maintaining personal hygiene standards

Avoid cross-infection   If you think about the sorts of things that you might handle during the day, then you will know why your hands can harbour harmful bacteria. Anything that comes into contact with the client's skin must be clean and hygienic, and this goes for your personal standards of health and hygiene too. You must prevent the risk of cross-infection and help your team to maintain a healthy, safe environment.

You must also take care of your hands to prevent developing **dermatitis**. Contact dermatitis is an occupational disease that can affect your hands; it creates a painful, itching sensation accompanied with a reddening and cracking of the skin.

Notice when things are running low

Shampoos and conditioners are in continual use and may need refilling throughout the day. Keep checking the levels of product. Notice the difference in weight between a full shampoo or conditioner bottle and one that is nearly empty. Do not wait until they have run out; fill them as required.

When you refill a product, unscrew the pump dispenser and wash it well to remove any dried-on product. Always use shampoo and conditioners sparingly; they are expensive, professional products and a small amount goes a long way. Wasting product will reduce business profits.

Preparing to shampoo checklist:

◆ Prepare the client with a clean fresh gown and towel.

◆ Make sure the client is comfortable and the position of the basin is correct.

◆ Brush through the hair carefully to remove any tangles and look for any signs of infection, infestation or injury that would stop you from carrying out the service.

◆ Ask the stylist what products you should use.

◆ Get the products ready and close at hand.

> **TOP TIP**
>
> Water is essential to all the salon's services, and shampooing alone can take 5–10 litres for each shampoo. Make sure that you always use water sparingly and never leave the taps running between shampoos, even if it is 'just' the cold water!

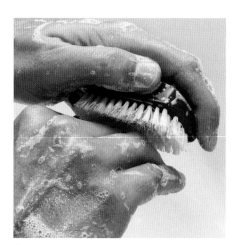

Ensure hands and nails are clean to avoid cross-infection

> **ACTIVITY**
>
> Answer the following questions in your portfolio:
>
> 1   Why is your posture important when you are shampooing and conditioning?
> 2   What safety considerations do you have to think about whilst the client is at the basin?
> 3   Why do you have to rinse the hair well after shampooing or conditioning?
> 4   Why do you need to keep the wash area clean and tidy?

> **TOP TIP**
>
> Keep an eye on the clock – remember that the stylist will need the client back in the styling chair as soon as possible so that they do not overrun or make the client late. Typically, a shampoo and simple surface conditioner should take 3–5 minutes.

Shampooing the client

ACTIVITY

Shampooing processes can differ between salons. What is the preferred process for shampooing in your salon, and how long should it take?

HEALTH & SAFETY

Raising the client too quickly from the basin can be dangerous. It may make some people feel dizzy when they try to stand up. If they have had any neck problems, it could cause injury. Make sure that you do not apply too much pressure on the back of the neck or joggle the client's head by wrongly applying uneven pressure on either side. Always test the water temperature on the back of your hands before transferring the flow to the client's head. Look out for changes and fluctuations in water temperature and pressure.

Some conditioning processes need heat to help them to penetrate more deeply. See Chapter 2 relating to the preparation and maintenance of hood dryers and **steamers**.

Types of shampoo

There are many different types of shampoo. The table describes some of the more popular types and their effects.

Type	Effects on the hair
Aloe vera	A popular, mild natural base ideal for healthy hair and scalps that can be used on a frequent basis
Chamomile	Better on greasy hair; has a natural lightening effect
Clarifying	Strong, deep acting; often used prior to chemical services to remove build-up of styling products and dirt
Coconut	Contains an emollient, which helps dry hair to regain its smoothness and elasticity
Jojoba	A natural base; better on normal to drier hair types
Lemon	Contains citric acid; ideal for greasy hair types or for removing product build-up
Medicated	Helps to maintain the normal state of the hair and scalp; contains antiseptics such as juniper or tea tree oil
Mint	A natural base suited to normal to slightly greasy hair, often used as a frequent use shampoo
Oil	Can contain a range of natural bases such as pine, palm and almond; these are used to smooth and soften drier hair and scalps
Soya	Helps to lock in moisture for the hair and scalp
Tea tree oil	A natural essential oil, which is like an antiseptic and will fight infections on the scalp

Following the stylist's instructions

Choosing the right products for the type of hair or following services is very important. If the wrong shampoo is used, the hair might become difficult to handle, fly-away, static, brittle or dull. Similarly, when the hair is to be permed or coloured and the shampoo does not remove the styling products from the hair, they might block the action of the chemicals in the technical service and interfere with the overall expected result.

Always ask the stylist what products you should use, get them ready and keep them to hand throughout the process.

How many times do I shampoo?

◆ Longer hair often requires two shampoos in order to develop a good lather, whereas short hair will often lather well with just one shampoo.

◆ Oilier, greasy hair usually needs at least two shampoos because it takes longer for the detergent in the shampoo to emulsify the grease and release it from the hair.

◆ Drier hair types can often be difficult to moisten and may also need two shampoos.

ACTIVITY

Answer the following questions in your portfolio:

1 How long should it take to complete the shampoo and conditioning service at work?
2 What is dermatitis and how do you avoid contracting it?
3 What types of protective wear are available for clients while they are in the salon?
4 How would you know which shampoo to use on a client?
5 Why is it important to keep checking the water temperature during shampooing?
6 Why should you turn the water off between shampoos?

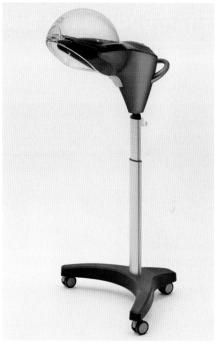

A steamer uses moist heat to help the conditioner penetrate

pH balance

The natural acid mantle of skin and hair has a pH balance of 5.5. Conditioners can be used to help rebalance the pH levels of hair to their natural slightly acidic value, particularly after chemical processes such as perming and colouring.

You may be familiar with the term pH balanced and think that you have seen it applied to other things as well. Well, it does occur in beauty products as well as hair, or you might have heard of it in advertising too.

Our skin is a complex organ that protects our bodies from infection and disease. It does this by being slightly acidic. This very mildly acidic value of pH 5.5 is just enough to prevent the rapid reproduction of harmful bacteria. If our skin were neutral, i.e. pH 7 which is neither acid nor alkaline, then the bacteria would grow and reproduce very quickly causing all sorts of infections and diseases.

So, all skin and hair care products are pH balanced and designed to match our skin's natural pH levels. This ensures that they are safe and hygienic to use.

TOP TIP

If you have any difficulties with the shampooing and conditioning process or any equipment that you are using, ask the stylist for assistance.

TOP TIP

Always check with the client to make sure that the water temperature is comfortable and not too hot for them before you begin shampooing.

Shampooing the client (Continued...)

Using the correct massage techniques

Three massage techniques are used in shampooing: **effleurage**, **rotary** and **friction**. A fourth technique, **petrissage**, is used during conditioning.

- Effleurage is a light, stroking movement applied with either the fingers or the palms of the hands. It is applied with an even, rhythmical movement with very little pressure, to induce a feeling of relaxation.

- Rotary is a circulatory movement made by the fingertips and thumbs with the hands in a loose 'claw-like' holding position. It is applied with even pressure on either side of the head, working from the sides above the ears backwards, over the back of the head and down into the nape of the neck. The rubbing process activates the shampoo, forming a rich lather and can be repeated until the hair is clean.

- Friction is a firmer, faster rubbing action made by the fingertips with the hands again in a loose 'claw-like' position. Friction is used for certain hair and scalp conditions or otherwise requested by the client for a more vigorous shampooing experience.

- Petrissage is a kneading movement of the skin that lifts and compresses underlying structures of the skin. The pressure applied should be intermittent and light, although firm enough to invigorate the part being treated.

Use effleurage massage to relax the client during shampooing

Controlling the water flow and temperature

During shampooing, control the water pressure to make sure that it is fast enough to rinse the hair properly, but slow enough so that it does not spray the client's face. Check the water temperature regularly by running the water over and between your fingers whilst you are rinsing. This way you will be able to gauge any fluctuations in temperature.

Use rotary massage technique to cleanse the hair and scalp

Rinsing and finishing off

After you have completed the shampoo(s), remove all traces of lather from the hair and scalp. If any residue remains, it could cause irritation and prevent further services from working properly. Check that the hair is rinsed well by running your fingers through the hair as if you were separating it and feeling for slight greasiness. Well-rinsed hair should feel squeaky clean and have some form of resistance between your fingers. After checking the hair, carefully remove the excess water by gently squeezing. The hair is now ready for conditioning.

TOP TIP

Hard rubbing and uneven pressure during rotary massage are uncomfortable for the client. Practise the right pressure with your colleagues at the salon.

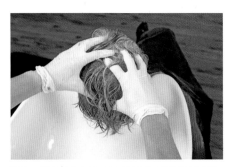

Use petrissage massage to invigorate the scalp

ACTIVITY

Construct a table in your portfolio with the following headings: 'Shampooing product', 'Who is the manufacturer?', 'What hair type is it for?', 'What does the product do?'. Then for each shampoo that your salon uses at the basin, complete the missing information. Use as many rows as you need.

STEP-BY-STEP: SHAMPOOING

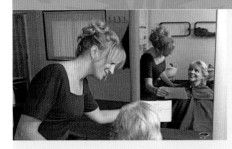

1 Sit the client at the styling station, put on a clean fresh gown and towel and discuss client's requirements.

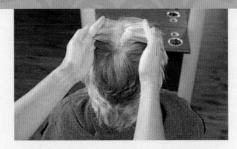

2 Check the hair and scalp prior to any treatment. Comb through the hair thoroughly. Take the client to the basin and prepare your products and equipment.

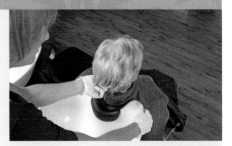

3 Adjust the basin to tilt the client's head back, ensure their position is comfortable. Position the towel so it protects the client but doesn't get wet.

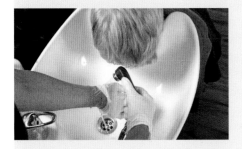

4 Turn on the water and adjust the temperature and pressure to suit the client's needs. Check the water temperature on the inside of your arm.

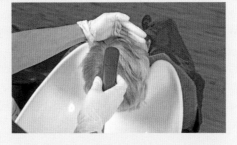

5 Carefully place a hand across the client's front hairline, 'damming' the water from splashing forward onto the face. Start rinsing the hair from the forehead.

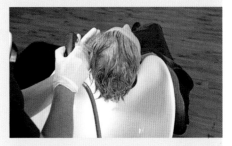

6 Dampen all the hair down both sides, remembering to cup over the ears until all the hair is wet.

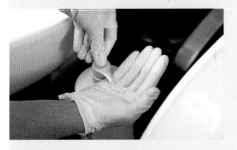

7 Apply a fifty pence amount of the correct shampoo to the palms of your hand.

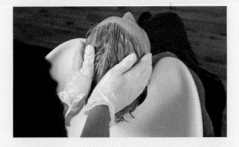

8 Lightly rub your hands together and apply the shampoo evenly all over the client's hair using a stroking movement. This massage technique is known as effleurage.

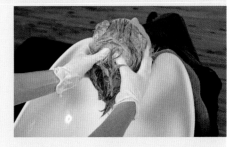

9 With the tips of your fingers massage the shampoo into the whole of the scalp with firm circular movements. This massage technique is known as rotary.

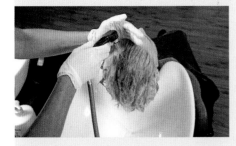

10 Rinse the hair thoroughly, checking the shampoo has been removed. Make sure that the client is shielded from the spray.

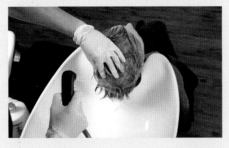

11 Repeat steps 5 to 9 and repeat the shampoo if necessary.

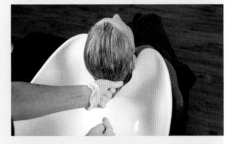

12 After shampooing, squeeze out excess moisture from the hair ready for the conditioner.

Conditioning the client's hair

Before you apply a conditioner

You must always ask the stylist before applying conditioner to the client's hair to ensure that it will not affect any following services. Conditioner will put a thin, laminating layer on the outside of the hair, and although this improves detangling and handling, it can be a barrier for some other chemical processes. For example, if you have shampooed in preparation for perming, a conditioner could prevent even penetration of the perming lotion and this could affect the overall perm result.

What are the benefits of using conditioners?

One of the main roles for hairdressers is to improve and maintain the condition of their clients' hair. If the cuticle surface of the client's hair is roughened or damaged, the appearance will be dull. Clients want their hair to shine, so we have to improve the surface by 'filling in' the missing or damaged areas of cuticle in order to make it as smooth as possible. We do this with help from conditioners. Conditioners make the hair easier to manage, easier to comb and easier to brush. Professional products protect and improve different hair types and disorders.

The main benefits of using a conditioner:

◆ Smoothes the cuticle edges.

◆ Improves handling and combing when the hair is both wet and dry.

◆ Temporarily repairs and fills damaged sites along the hair shaft or missing areas of the cuticle or cortex.

◆ Provides shine, lustre and sheen.

◆ Creates flexibility and movement by locking in moisture.

◆ Re-balances the pH value of the hair to a slightly acid 5.5.

Types of conditioner

There are two types of conditioners: **surface conditioners** and **penetrating (treatment) conditioners**.

◆ Surface conditioners work on the surface of the hair. Their main purpose is to coat the cuticle layer of the hair and improve handling by making it easier to comb through. Surface conditioners improve the hair's look and feel by adding shine and moisture.

◆ Penetrating conditioners penetrate deeper into the hair. Their main purpose is to enter the cortex through the damaged areas of cuticle and to fill the air spaces caused by chemical or thermal damage. They replenish the moisture levels within the hair to make it flexible and elastic, add shine and improve handling.

Some conditioning rinses are used after perms and chemical straighteners as antioxidants (**antioxidant conditioners**) to stop any further oxidation or to balance pH (**pH balance conditioners**).

TOP TIP

Wet hair can tangle easily, which makes it very painful to comb through. Therefore, when combing through wet hair, always start at the nape. Disentangle the ends first, then work back up through the lengths getting closer to the scalp.

ACTIVITY

Construct a table in your portfolio with the following headings: 'Conditioning product', 'Who is the manufacturer?', 'What hair type is it for?', 'What does the product do?'. Then for each conditioner that your salon uses at the basin, complete the missing information. Use as many rows as you need.

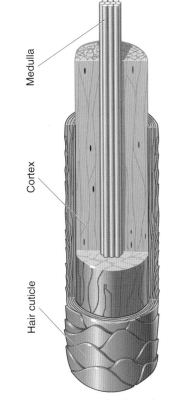

These images show the external surface and a cross-section through the hair. Notice that the 'free' edges of the cuticle point towards the points of the hair.

ACTIVITY

Self-assessment for shampooing and conditioning

Copy the following statements into your portfolio and put a tick or cross beside each one to show how much you have learnt. When you have completed it ask your supervisor to sign and date it.

1   I know what the effleurage movement is and when to use this massage technique.

2   I know what the rotary movement is and when to use this massage technique.

3   I know what the friction movement is and when to use this massage technique.

4   I know what the petrissage movement is and when to use this massage technique.

5   I know why and how to detangle clients' hair properly.

6   I know how to dispense the right amount of shampoo product for a client.

7   I know how to dispense the right amount of conditioning product for a client.

8   I can regulate the water pressure and temperature properly.

Conditioning

Each conditioning treatment is specific to the task in hand. It is therefore extremely important to follow the manufacturer's instructions so that the product can do its job. More damaged types of hair require the assistance of heat from a hood dryer or a steamer for deeper penetration. The following sequence provides guidelines for applying a general surface conditioner.

STEP-BY-STEP: CONDITIONING

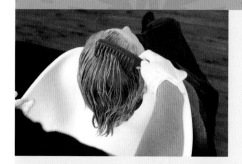
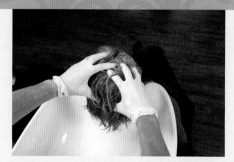
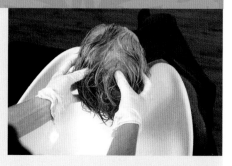

1 Apply a fifty pence size amount of conditioner into the palm of your hand and apply the conditioner to the client's hair using effleurage massage movements. On longer hair more conditioner should be applied and combed through using a wide tooth comb to detangle the hair. Start at the ends of the client's hair and work up to the roots.

2 Use the pads of your fingers in firm slow, circular movements to lift and rotate the scalp. This massage technique is called petrissage. Start at the front top of the head and work down to the nape.

3 Repeat this circular process several times. Allow the client to relax and the conditioner to smooth the hair cuticles. This step should take approximately three or four minutes.

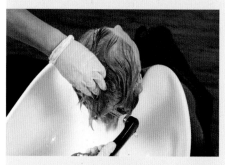
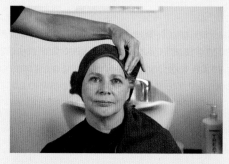
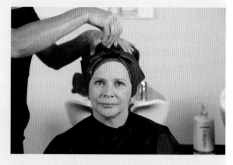

4 When the process is complete, rinse away all the excess product from the hair while remembering to shield the client's face and make-up if they are wearing any.

5 Remove PPE and come to the side of the client. Sit the client up and use the towel around their shoulders to wrap the hair.

6 Carefully envelope the hair in a clean towel and move the client to the styling section for detangling.

TOP TIP

When detangling during or after conditioning, always comb the hair from points to roots.

CourseMate video: Shampooing and conditioning

SUMMARY

Now you have finished this chapter you should have a clearer picture of all the essential aspects associated with shampooing and conditioning. In particular, you should now have a good understanding and be able to:

✓ prepare the client adequately for a range of backwash processes

✓ describe how shampooing and conditioning processes work

✓ carry out shampooing services for a range of clients with differing needs

✓ carry out conditioning treatments for a range of clients with differing needs.

In addition, you will understand how these processes will enable you to work more efficiently and effectively in daily salon routines.

REVISION QUESTIONS

Q1.   Copy and complete this sentence: Shampooing cleans hair by _____ dirt, skin scale and product build-up.

Fill in the blank

Q2.   Conditioning treatments raise the hair cuticle?

True or false?

Q3.   By which of the following methods do conditioners work on the hair?
(You may choose more than one answer.)

attraction	☐ a
repulsion	☐ b
erosion	☐ c
absorption	☐ d
friction	☐ e
propulsion	☐ f

Q4.   Shampoos contain bleach?

True or false?

Q5.   The detergent in shampoo lifts grease off hair by suspending it in water. What is this called? (Choose one answer.)

hydrophobic	○ a
hydrophilic	○ b
emulsion	○ c
erosion	○ d

7 Styling and Finishing Hair

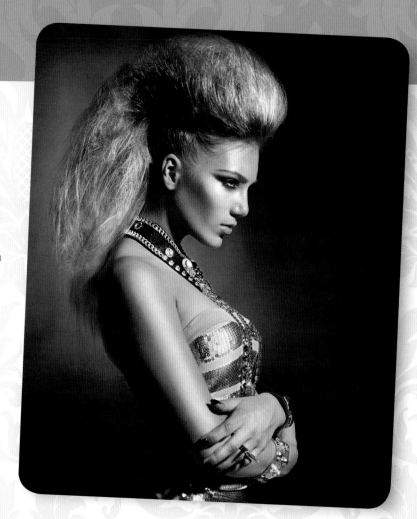

LEARNING OBJECTIVES

When you have finished this chapter you should:

◆ be able to blow-dry hair into style

◆ be able to work safely at all times

◆ know the range of tools and products used in styling and finishing hair

◆ understand the basic science related to blow-drying

◆ know your salon's standards and expectations for styling clients' hair

◆ be able to communicate professionally and provide aftercare advice.

KEY TERMS

alpha keratin

beta keratin

cool shot

cortex

cuticle

humidity

medulla

polypeptide chains

polypeptides

INFORMATION COVERED IN THIS CHAPTER

PRACTICAL SKILLS

Learn how to work safely at all times when providing the service to clients.

Learn how to prepare the client and their hair correctly for the service.

Learn how to use both flat brushes and round brushes for styling hair into shape.

Learn how to use heated styling equipment safely when finishing hair.

UNDERPINNING KNOWLEDGE

Know how to use styling products for blow-drying and finishing hair.

Understand the basic science related to blow-drying and heat styling.

Know the salon and legal requirements in relation to blow-drying.

Know how to use blow-drying tools and the techniques for using them.

Know how to communicate effectively and professionally.

INTRODUCTION

Blow-drying has been the most popular styling technique for finishing clients' hair for many years. Its popularity has grown as it provides the main styling option for people to manage themselves at home. The effects can be achieved quickly and easily, and people are far more aware now of the damage that can be caused to their hair by the incorrect use of heat-styling equipment.

This chapter covers all the things associated with this service. You will be learning how to style hair with different types of brushes and heated equipment and also the products that can be used to help create the desired effects and maintain healthy hair.

Preparing for the service

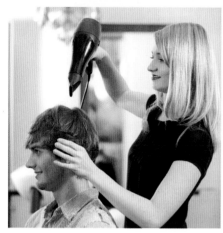

The position of your client and your standing position are equally important to avoid fatigue and back problems

Correctly protect and position clients and yourself

Before you can start a blow-dry the hair must be shampooed, so the client will have wet hair when they arrive at the styling unit. The first thing you need to do is make sure that if the towel is taken away the client's hair will not drip. This is part of good customer care, especially if the client has long hair.

Check that the client's gown is still secure, then remove excess moisture by gently squeezing the hair in the towel or by light rubbing. After finishing with the damp towel put a clean, dry, fresh towel around the shoulders and secure it with a clip. Then take a wide-tooth comb and work through the ends of the hair to remove tangles near the points. Work back up through the lengths, combing as you go, until the hair combs freely without knots.

Work position   Salon chairs are designed with comfort and safety in mind. Your client's back should be flat against the back of the chair and the chair at a comfortable height for you to work. Do not be afraid to ask the client to sit up. If the client slouches, their head and neck will be at an angle that makes your job of styling almost impossible, and this poor posture could cause them back pain and possible injury.

Your posture   As a stylist or barber your standing position is equally important to avoid injury. Stand close enough to the styling chair so that you stand upright when either working from:

◆ a side of the chair position – so as to not raise your arms above shoulder height at any time during the service to avoid pain and muscle fatigue

◆ a back of the chair position – the mirror in front of you, with a clear view of the client's head to see the shape of their hair as you are styling.

TOP TIP

You want to start on the right foot and give the client a professional image of you and what you are about to do.

Keeping the work area clean and safe to use at all times

Prepare any equipment or styling products that you need beforehand. Prepare your trolley if you use one as a workstation. Remove all items and previously used materials from the shelves before any client sits at the styling unit, including:

◆ combs, brushes and sectioning clips

◆ mugs, cups and saucers

◆ magazines, papers, etc.

◆ styling and finishing products.

The work space should be tidy; working surfaces should be cleaned with a disinfecting spray and the mirror polished. The whole work area should be hygienic and give the client a positive and professional image.

For more information on cleaning and salon maintenance, see Chapter 2 Preparing for work.

Maintaining personal hygiene standards

All the materials that come into contact with the client's skin and hair must be clean and hygienic. Similarly, your own personal standards of health and hygiene should not present any risk to the client. This will prevent the risk of cross-infection and helps to maintain a healthy, safe environment.

Using tools and equipment safely

All the tools that you use must be hygienic and safe for use. They must be cleaned and sterilized before they can be used on the client.

Completing the service efficiently

However much fun doing a blow-dry may seem, remember to keep to time:

◆ Do not make the client late as they may have other plans that day.

◆ Do not make the stylist run late – they may need to alter your blow-dry afterwards and have other waiting clients.

◆ Remain professional – if you are given responsibility it must be up to standard.

This table provides a guideline for how long each type of blow-dried style will take:

Hair length	Style	Brush	Time
short	straight	Denman or vented	20 minutes
mid-length, bob	straight	Denman or vented	25 minutes
long, one length	straight	large round	35 minutes
Short	volume and lift or curly	small round	25 minutes
mid-length, layered	movement and texture	medium round	30 minutes
long, layered	movement and texture	large round and medium round	40 minutes
medium, layered	curly	small round	35 minutes
long, layered	curly	medium round and small round	45 minutes

> For more information on preventing infection, personal health and hygiene, see Chapter 3 Health and safety.

ACTIVITY

Different salons have different ways of doing things. Find out what your salon's policy is regarding:

◆ preparing the client prior to styling

◆ preparing tools and equipment ready for use

◆ the use of styling products within the salon

◆ retail products and how they are brought up in conversation with the client.

Make sure that you always:

✓ wash your hands before attending to any clients

✓ wear minimal jewellery so that it doesn't dangle or tangle in the client's hair

✓ wear comfortable (flatter and not open-toed) footwear when on the salon floor

✓ are aware of bad breath – use breath fresheners if you have a problem

✓ take a shower daily before going to work

✓ make sure your workwear is clean and fresh every day

✓ think how you want to be seen by others – you are an advertisement for the service you offer, so make sure that your hair is clean and styled

✓ minimize the risk of cross-infection to your colleagues and clients.

TOP TIP

Always follow the stylist's instructions for completing the hairstyle. Don't just do what you feel will be right – it might be wrong.

Basic hair science

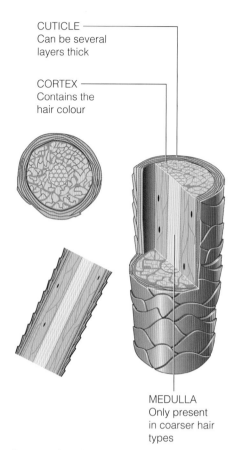

CUTICLE
Can be several
layers thick

CORTEX
Contains the
hair colour

MEDULLA
Only present
in coarser hair
types

Cross section of hair

If we look at the basic structure of hair in the diagram below we can see that there are three distinctly different layers.

The cuticle

The **cuticle** is the outer layer of colourless cells that form the protective surface of the hair. Properties of the cuticle:

◆ It regulates the chemicals entering and damaging the hair and protects the hair from excessive heat and drying.

◆ Cells overlap like tiles on a roof with the free edges pointing towards the tips of the hair.

◆ Has layers that affect the hair texture – hair with fewer layers of cuticle is finer than coarser hair types, which have several layers.

◆ In good condition is tightly closed and resists the entry of moisture, e.g. when shampooing, or hairdressing chemicals when colouring or perming.

◆ In poor condition will be dry or porous and have damaged or missing cuticle layers; this allows moisture and chemicals to saturate and overload the hair.

◆ In good condition will allow the hair to dry more quickly than damaged, porous hair because porous hair absorbs moisture and will take longer to dry.

◆ Temporary colours coat the cuticles, making the hair look a different colour.

◆ Semi-permanent colours coat the outside and penetrate to some of the lower layers to make the hair look a different colour.

◆ Surface conditioners coat the cuticle to add moisture, shine and increase the hair's flexibility.

Hair in good condition has a smooth, flat cuticle layer, tightly closed along the hair shaft with the free edges pointing towards the ends of the hair. Hair in poor condition has a raised cuticle; the edges are not flat and feel roughened. This can expose the cortex below, making the hair very dry and damaged.

The cortex

The **cortex** is the middle and largest layer. It is made up of long 'rope-like' fibres twisted together. Inside these fibres are long, spiralled structures called **polypeptides**. The properties of the cortex:

◆ It forms the largest part or area of the hair.

◆ All permanent hairdressing chemical processes take place within the cortex.

◆ Hair strength is directly related to the condition of the cortex.

◆ Hair elasticity is directly proportional to the condition of the cortex.

◆ Naturally occurring colour pigments (pheomelanin and eumelanin) are scattered throughout the cortex to give hair its natural colour appearance.

◆ Artificial colours such as quasi-permanent and permanent colours are deposited within it during chemical processing to create a new and different appearance.

◆ Condition and quality of the hair is related to the condition of the cortex.

◆ Hair lighteners react with the natural hair pigments to make the hair appear lighter.

◆ Penetrating conditioning treatments help to 'lock in' moisture in order to improve the condition or rebuild the cortex structure.

The medulla

The medulla is the central, inner part of the hair. Properties of the medulla:

◆ It only exists in medium to coarser hair types.

◆ It is often intermittent in different parts throughout the length.

◆ Is not involved in hairdressing services, chemical processes or treatments.

Alpha and beta keratin – the principles of heat styling (the temporary set)

Hair that has been shampooed and left to dry naturally is known as alpha keratin, or in its alpha keratin state. When you shampoo hair and then dry it into style, stretching it with a brush, it is called beta keratin. This will go back to alpha keratin when the hair is moistened, perhaps by moisture in the air such as a 'steamy' bathroom.

This is the principle of heated styling and the reason why hair stays in a blow-dried or set position. On the following page we look at the tiny spiral structures within the cortex called polypeptide chains.

Before hair is shampooed, the hydrogen bonds hold the polypeptide chains close together. Hair in this natural un-stretched state is called alpha keratin.

After shampooing, many of the hydrogen bonds are broken. This allows the hair to be stretched around a roller or brush.

During styling the hair is stretched, dried and allowed to cool into the new shape. The hair is now in a beta keratin state. Here we can see that the hydrogen bonds are reformed in new positions on the polypeptide chains.

The hair will stay in this new (beta keratin) shape until it is made wet or absorbs moisture from the atmosphere. (You will notice how both sets and blow-dries drop very quickly in wet, misty or foggy weather.)

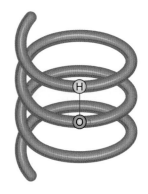

Alpha keratin:
dry hair unstretched

Alpha keratin

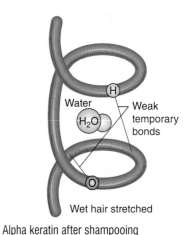

Water
Weak temporary bonds
H_2O

Wet hair stretched

Alpha keratin after shampooing

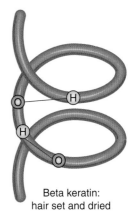

Beta keratin:
hair set and dried

Beta keratin

ACTIVITY

Draw a diagram to show the basic structure of the hair. On the diagram show the positions of the cuticle, cortex and medulla, and indicate the root ends of the hair and the points of the hair. Now answer the following questions in your portfolio:

1. What are alpha and beta keratin?
2. What does the cuticle layer look like?
3. What are the indicators of hair in good condition?
4. What are the indicators of hair in poor condition?

5. What effect does humidity have on a finished hairstyle?
6. What is another name for a round brush?
7. Give two examples of flat brushes.

Blow-dry hair

Following the stylist's instructions

Although you are styling the client's hair, the stylist is ultimately responsible for what you do; therefore, you must follow their instructions. Use only the tools and sequence as they instruct you to. For instance, if they have specifically said that they want the back of the client's one length bob sectioned off, and the underneath dried first, then that is where you must start. The stylist will provide you with the instructions required for a satisfactory result in the time available. If you make any changes you will probably go wrong and possibly be left with an unhappy client. If you start struggling, ask the stylist for help.

When you finish the style the client may ask for some finishing products like wax, defining crème, moulding clay or hairspray. Do not apply these products unless you have been told to by the stylist.

> **TOP TIP**
>
> If the hair is long you will need to work from the V points, through the lengths and back up towards the roots because the ends will always be wetter than the root area.

Applying the products correctly

Always try to minimize waste – use care and control when you dispense the products and only use as much as you need. Excess product:

◆ will either be thrown away or rubbed off into a towel

◆ could overload the scalp area and irritate the client's scalp.

Applying styling products   Always use styling products sparingly. The following images show how much mousse should be applied to short- to medium-length hair:

> **TOP TIP**
>
> Do not overload the hair with product unless the style/client requires it. This will make the hair unpleasantly hard and you may have to re-shampoo and start over.

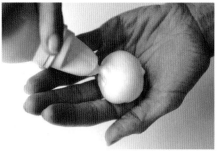

Standard styling mousse to be applied to the mid-lengths and ends.

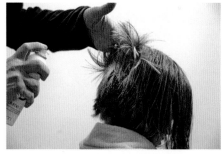

Root/volumizing mousse being applied to root area by separating the hair and spraying at different points where volume is required.

Applying finishing products

Hairspray fixes hair into shape. Always hold the can upright and at least 30cm away from the hair. Make sure that the pinhole in the nozzle faces the client's hair and lightly mist for a few seconds.

Moulding/defining crème adds texture and hold. It is ideal for adding texture to layered hairstyles. Take a small amount of product onto the end of your index finger. Transfer this to your inner fingers on both hands evenly and then work into the outer layers to create the textured effect. Add more to create the desired effect.

Serum provides control and shine, and smooths down frizzes. This product is available as light hair oils or moisturizing control crèmes. Apply a couple of drops to the fingers and work together between the fingers on both hands. Apply carefully and evenly throughout the lengths to improve the look and feel of the hair.

Gel provides a strong, wet-look hold in any hair type. It is ideal for adding strong, spiky texture to layered hairstyles. To use, take a small amount of product onto the ends of your fingers. Transfer this to the fingers of both hands evenly and then work into the outer layers to create the textural effect. Add more to create the sculpted effect.

Wax provides strong, medium or soft hold in any textured hairstyle. Take a small amount of product onto the end of your index finger. Transfer this to your fingertips on both hands evenly and then work into the outer hair. Add more to create the textured effect.

> **TOP TIP**
> Always follow the manufacturer's instructions when handling styling and finishing products.

> **TOP TIP**
> Use products sparingly. You can always add more as you need it. Do not apply too much at first.

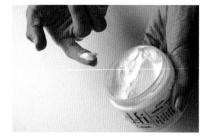
Take a small amount of moulding crème onto the tip of your index finger

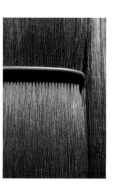
Use serum for smooth control and better conditioning

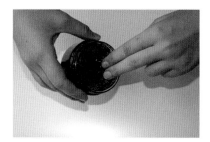
Gel provides a strong, wet look

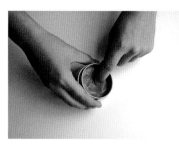
Wax provides strong, medium or light hold in any textured hairstyle

Blow-dry hair (Continued...)

Product	What is it for?	How is it applied?	When do you use it?
Styling mousse	a general styling aid for adding volume and providing hold	blob the size of a small orange evenly to the lengths	on dampened hair before sectioning and drying
Root lift mousse	a special mousse that has a directional nozzle, allowing you to apply foam at or near to the roots	lift and separate sections of dampened hair so that the root area is exposed; hold the can so that the nozzle aims the foam near the root	on hair that needs body but doesn't require setting hold at the mid-lengths and points
Styling gel/glaze	a wet look, firm hold finish on shorter hair styles	small 'pea-sized' amount from the fingertips all over evenly (you can always add more if necessary)	not easy to blow-dry, can be used in finger drying and scrunch-dry techniques
Moulding clay	a dual purpose product for styling or finishing that bonds the hair with firm hold	on damp hair – a small 'pea-sized' amount from the fingertips all over evenly; on dry hair – with fingertips to the points of the hair for texture and definition	a firm textural bond on most lengths of hair
Defining crème	a finishing product that provides control on unruly hair	on dry hair: small 'droplet' amounts a little at a time with fingertips	throughout the lengths of the hair for smooth control and conditioning
Defining wax	a slightly greasy finishing product that provides textural effects on short to longer hair	on dry hair: apply small 'pea-sized' amounts a little at a time with fingertips	throughout the ends of the hair for style definition and/or texture effects
Serum	a slightly oily finishing product that provides improved handling and shine	on dry hair: small droplet amounts a little at a time with fingertips	throughout the lengths of the hair for smooth control and better conditioning
Hairspray	a finishing product in a variety of holds/strengths, pump or aerosol spray	mist hair from about 30–40cm away from the hair for a 'fixed' hold on dry hair	final fixative, overall sealer or a scrunching, textural finish
Dry wax	a non-greasy finishing product that provides textural effects on short to longer hair	on dry hair: small 'pea-sized' amounts a little at a time with fingertips	used throughout the ends of the hair for style definition and/or textural effects

ACTIVITY

Product knowledge

For each of the products listed below, find out which sorts of hairstyles they are most appropriate for. Try to find examples of these in style magazines or from websites on the Internet. Copy and complete the table in your portfolio.

Product	Suitable styles and lengths
Soft wax	
Gel	
Moulding clay	
Serum	
Mousse	
Hard wax	

TOP TIP

The way that you approach the work will say a lot about your levels of ability to the client. Be confident, be careful, but above all be professional.

Maintaining the client's comfort

Always check with the client to see that they are comfortable throughout the service. Mind how you use the dryer and direct the heat over the surface of the brush when blow-drying. If the blast of heat and air deflects off the edge that is nearest the client's scalp you will burn them. They will be annoyed and you will look foolish, and they will have lost any confidence in you!

TOP TIP

Moisture will naturally fall and run down the hair shaft with gravity, so starting near the root area will always quicken the drying process. After a couple of passes through the hair, the section will be dry.

Using brushes to style hair professionally

These images show the correct position of the dryer nozzle in relation to both the brush and the direction of the heat.

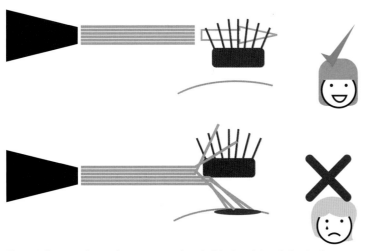

HEALTH & SAFETY

Avoid cross-infection and cross-infestation: always use cleaned and sterilized brushes on the clients.

The top diagram shows the correct angle to hold a brush in relation to the client's head. The heat from a wrongly positioned brush (bottom diagram) will burn the client within 2–3 seconds, regardless of heat setting or speed used.

Blow-dry hair (Continued...)

Drying the hair – roots to points

You should only work on small sections, no larger than the surface area of the brush you are using. If the sections are too large you will not be able to dry each mesh of hair properly. This will affect how long the blow-dry lasts. Be careful not to overheat any sections of the hair while you are drying, as it will damage the hair.

Start the blow-dry at the lower back. Section any surplus out of the way and secure it with a clip. Then, taking your dryer in one hand, offer the dryer across to the section to check the angle of the nozzle. The air should be parallel to the angle of the hair. Take your brush in the other hand and introduce the bristles to the hair near the root area. Pick up and turn the brush so that the hair is caught across the bristles. Turn on the dryer and, now aiming across the brush, follow the brush downwards with the dryer, holding it about 10–15cm away.

Focusing the jet stream

The hair can only dry if the blast from the dryer is working over the surface of it. So carefully aim the flat, jet stream of heated air across the surface of the brush, shielding the heat from the back (scalp) side of the brush. As you move the brush down, move the dryer down so that it *mirrors* the position of the brush at always the same distance away. Blow-drying from root to point ensures that the cuticle lies flat, reducing flyaway frizz and smoothing the overall result.

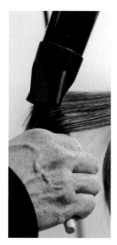

See how the brush is held in relation to the blow-dryer

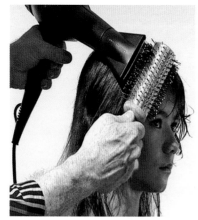

See how the brush is held in relation to the client's head

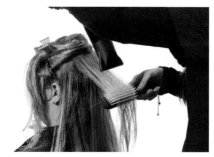

Maintain an even tension upon the hair as you work through each section. Be careful not to overheat any sections of the hair while you are drying

TOP TIP

Never try to dry saturated hair. You need to work with hair that is damp rather than wet, so dry off the hair in the areas that need it first, using a clean dry towel. You can always re-moisten the hair if it becomes too dry.

If you are using a round, radial brush you will find that you need to take a section and wind the hair around the brush. Again, focus the jet stream over the curved surfaces of the brush, but this time from both sides. This will enable the hair to dry around the brush, forming part of the wave. Then after drying and while still warm, use a **cool shot** from the dryer (or use 'blast only' without heat settings) to 'freeze' the wave into place. (This fixes the style with more durability, as in setting – when rollers are allowed to cool down before removal and final brushing and dressing out.) If you do not allow the meshes of hair to cool, the result will be limp and will not last as long. Finally, with the section dry, you can take down another mesh, ready for drying into position.

Blow-dry styling dos and don'ts

Do	Don't
✓ Dry the hair well so that it is moist but not wet before starting the blow-dry.	✗ Don't leave damp towels around the client's shoulders.
✓ Take small sections that you can control and dry evenly throughout.	✗ Don't leave the dryer running whilst you re-section the hair.
✓ Direct the flow of air away from the client.	✗ Don't use the top heat setting unless it's really necessary.
✓ Adjust the chair height so you can reach the top of the client's head without over-stretching.	✗ Don't pass the brush to the client for them to hold in between sectioning.
✓ Ask the client to adjust their head position if you need to.	✗ Don't try to use the same hand for brush work on both sides of the head.
✓ Clip out of the way any sections that are not yet being worked on.	✗ Don't over-dry the hair as this will cause permanent damage.

TOP TIP

When finger-drying hair:

◆ always work with damp and not saturated hair – rough-dry if necessary

◆ work on small areas/sections of hair

◆ try to dry the hair in the direction of roots to points – it will dry more quickly and keep the cuticle layer smoother, making it look healthier and shinier

◆ avoid burning the scalp – angle your dryer away from the head

◆ move the position of your client's head in order to get around and cover all areas of the head

◆ use both hands to dry the hair – swap the dryer around as this enables you to work on both sides of the head effectively.

Finger-drying Finger-drying is a fast and more natural way of drying hair into style. After removing excess moisture from the hair, some mousse can be applied to provide some body and texture to work with. The main idea of finger-drying is to use a blow-dryer with the fingers in a directional drying process, on generally shorter hair. There are other benefits to drying hair this way:

◆ It allows a style to be moulded on hair that would normally be too short to dry with brushes.

◆ It can be used to style longer hair into cascades of curly movement, either on natural or permed hair.

Blow-dry hair (Continued...)

Working with tensioned hair   You have to maintain an even tension on the meshes of hair throughout the blow-drying service. This ensures that the hair will dry with a smooth, sleek effect without frizzed or crimped areas. If you do create a kinked, uneven result, you can lightly spray down with water and start again. Look out for the hair in the sectioning clips waiting to be dried too. If the hair has a natural tendency to wave or curl, it might disfigure before you can style it. Again, lightly mist it down with water and start over.

STEP-BY-STEP: SECTIONING THE HAIR

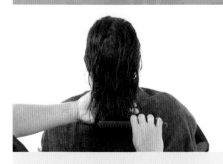

1 After shampooing and conditioning squeeze out any excess moisture and detangle the client's hair with a wide-toothed comb. Remember to comb from points to roots in the direction of the cuticle.

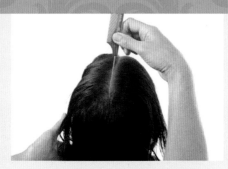

2 Using a pin-tail comb, draw one continuous line from the centre of the forehead to the base of the neck.

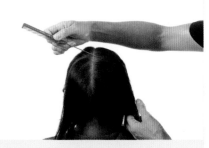

3 Pick up one side of the client's hair and brush it over to one side. Then draw another continuous straight line from the centre point of the top of the head.

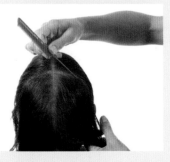

4 Continue to the top of the ear on one side then repeat on the other side.

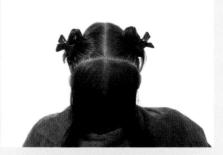

5 Twist and clip up the front sections in quarters with butterfly clips. You should have four identical neat sections.

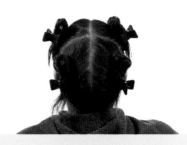

6 The head should be sectioned into quarters and look like a hot cross bun from the top.

TOP TIP

Sectioning is essential for applying penetrating conditioners, permanent colours, blow-drying and cutting. The neater the sectioning the easier it is to master all of the hairdressing techniques.

CourseMate video: Sectioning hair

STEP-BY-STEP: FLAT BRUSH BLOW-DRY ON LONGER HAIR

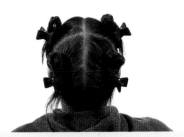

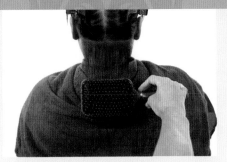

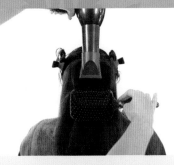

1 After shampooing and conditioning, section the hair into a hot cross bun with a pin-tail comb, securing with butterfly clips.

2 Using a pin-tail comb, take a 3cm horizontal section above the nape from the two back sections. Secure the remainder of the hair out of the way neatly.

3 Wrap the hair around your brush. Dry the hair with a nozzle attachment parallel to the hair from above. Work from roots to ends in the direction of the cuticle to leave a smooth frizz-free finish.

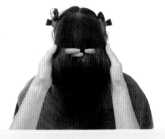

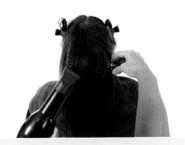

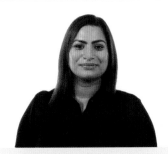

4 Make sure the section is completely dry before taking the next section. Work all the way up the back of the head using the same technique for drying the client's hair and then dry the sides following the same technique.

5 Be careful with the direction of the air from the dryer nozzle as it is easy to burn the client.

6 The finished look.

CourseMate video: Flat brush blow-dry

TOP TIP

As the hair gets longer you will need to dry the root area first before attempting to dry the ends.

Heated equipment: straightening irons and tongs

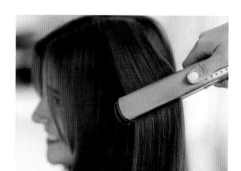

Ceramic straighteners are very effective at smoothing away frizz

Electric curling tongs, heated brushes and straightening irons are a popular way of applying finish to a hairstyle. They are particularly useful in situations where:

◆ setting or blow-drying will not achieve the desired look

◆ the hair is not in a suitable condition to be dried into shape.

Sometimes you will not achieve the result that you or the client is expecting. When extra volume, movement or curl is needed, heated tongs and/or brushes will provide a quick solution. They can be bought in a variety of different sizes (i.e. diameters and widths), which give different levels of movement and finish.

Professional heated tongs and straighteners have a thermostatic temperature control. This is particularly useful as you can 'dial up' the heat setting required to match the client's hair type. This reduces the risk of damage to the hair from excess heat.

Straightening irons and particularly ceramic straightening irons have been a very popular way of calming unruly hair. They work by electrically heating two parallel plates so that the hair can be run between them in one movement from roots to ends, smoothing out the unwanted wave or frizz in the process.

Ceramic straighteners have been particularly successful as they heat up in just a few moments and have a higher operating temperature than metal irons (180°–200°C). This alarmingly high temperature is potentially damaging to hair but, because they have the ability to transfer heat quickly and smoothly to the hair without grabbing, they are very effective in creating smoother effects. Nevertheless, because of their temperature you must check them before you introduce them to the hair so that you do not permanently damage the client's hair.

When straightening is needed to complement the look on longer hair, it is sometimes better to straighten each section as the blow-dry proceeds. If you start underneath, each section is completely finished before you move on up the head. The hair will stay flatter from the start and each section will be dry, stopping the hair from reverting to its previous state.

TOP TIP

Very hot styling tools without a non-slip coating or ceramic surface often tend to stick when they are introduced to hair that has styling products on it.

TOP TIP

Hot styling tools can make hair static and flyaway. Heat protection sprays control this and protect the hair from being excessively overheated.

Keeping the heated styling equipment clean

With prolonged use, the surfaces on tongs and straighteners can suffer from product build-up. This should always be looked for, as any residue of styling products such as wax, hairsprays and gels, serums, etc. will stick to the slippery, smooth surfaces and create roughened areas that will grab and lock on to the hair when they are hot. This is damaging as it will burn the hair.

STEP-BY-STEP: CREATING SPIRALLED CURLS WITH CERAMIC TONGS

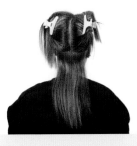

1 When your client is comfortably seated, section off and secure the hair at the nape.

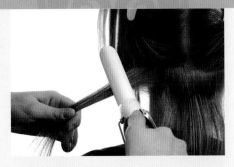

2 On your curling tongs, dial up the correct temperature for the hair type and place the barrel of the tongs near the root area and begin to turn.

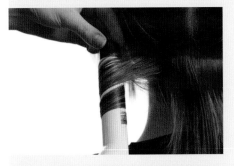

3 As you turn, slightly open and close the tongs so that hair is drawn into the barrel of the tongs. This produces an attractive spiral curl.

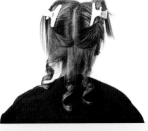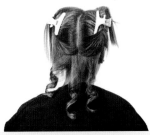

4 With the lower section done, carry on working up through the hair until the back area is complete. New warm curls are then gently laid over cooler, previously curled hair.

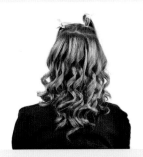

5 The back of the hair should start to look like this as you continue the same patterning technique in the side areas.

6 The finished look has texture and movement.

For more information on styling tools and equipment, sterilization and tool maintenance, see Chapter 2 Prepare for work.

HEALTH & SAFETY

Always check the condition of the lead and plug before attempting to plug the dryer into the mains socket. If it looks damaged or the cable is broken, tell your supervisor immediately.

Heated equipment: straightening irons and tongs (Continued...)

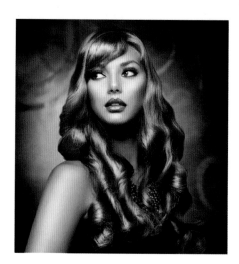

ACTIVITY

Product knowledge

Copy the table below into your portfolio. Then complete the missing information to show how and when the products are applied.

Product	How is it applied?	When is it applied?
Mousse		
Root mousse		
Styling gel		
Serum		
Defining crème		
Hair wax		

HEALTH & SAFETY

Points to remember when using heated styling equipment

◆ Never get too close to the client's head with hot styling equipment.

◆ Never leave the styling equipment on one area of hair for more than a few seconds.

◆ Always replace the styling tools into their holder at the workstation when not in use.

◆ Always check the filters on the back of hand dryers to make sure that they are not blocked (this will cause the dryer to overheat and possibly ignite).

◆ Look out for trailing flexes across the floor or around the back of styling chairs.

◆ Let tools cool down before putting them back into storage.

◆ Always check for damage or kinks in flexes or damaged plugs.

◆ Never use damaged equipment under any circumstances.

SUMMARY

Now you have finished this chapter you should have a clearer picture of all the essential aspects associated with styling and finishing hair. In particular, you should now have a good understanding and be able to:

✓ prepare the clients for styling and finishing services

✓ describe the effects that styling and finishing has on the hair structure

✓ know when to use and apply styling products during the service

✓ carry out the basic styling techniques involved in blow-drying and heat-styling using a variety of different tools and equipment.

In addition, you will understand how these processes will enable you to work more efficiently and effectively in daily salon routines.

REVISION QUESTIONS

Q1. Copy and complete this sentence: Brushes can be _____ by putting them into a UV cabinet.

Fill in the blank

Q2. A round brush is also called a radial brush

True or False

Q3. Which of the following are types of blow-drying brushes? (You may choose more than one answer.)

flat	☐	a
square	☐	b
oblong	☐	c
oval	☐	d
round	☐	e
triangular	☐	f

Q4. The bristles of brushes are normally made from plastics

True or False

Q5. What state is hair changed into during the process of blow-drying? (Choose one answer.)

alpha keratin	○	a
beta keratin	○	b
permanent set	○	c
damaged	○	d

8 Dressing, Plaiting and Twisting Hair

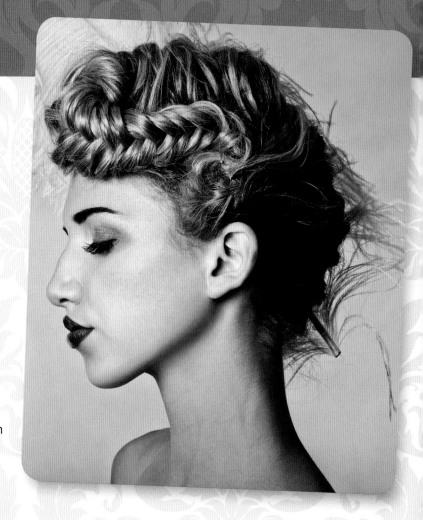

LEARNING OBJECTIVES

When you have finished this chapter you should:

◆ be able to style hair using different setting methods

◆ be able to dress hair using different techniques

◆ be able to style hair using different plaiting and twisting techniques

◆ know how to secure and fix hair into shape

◆ understand the physical changes within hair during styling

◆ know the range of tools and products used in styling and finishing hair

◆ be able to communicate professionally and provide aftercare advice.

KEY TERMS

back-brushing

braiding bands

cornrows

comb-out

fishtail plait

French plait

off-base rollering

on-base rollering

traction alopecia

wet setting

INFORMATION COVERED IN THIS CHAPTER

PRACTICAL SKILLS

Learn how to work safely at all times when providing the service to clients.

Learn how to prepare the client and their hair correctly for the service.

Learn how to use both wet and dry setting rollers.

Learn how to use heated styling equipment safely when finishing hair.

Learn how to create a variety of plaited and twisted effects.

Learn how to fix different hair lengths into style using grips, pins and clips.

UNDERPINNING KNOWLEDGE

Know how to use styling products for dressing and finishing hair.

Understand the basic science related to setting and heat styling.

Know the salon and legal requirements in relation to setting and dressing hair.

Know how to use setting, dressing and plaiting tools and equipment, and the techniques for using them.

Know how to communicate effectively and professionally.

INTRODUCTION

This chapter looks at the creative effects that can be achieved by dressing, plaiting and twisting hair. It incorporates a variety of techniques including setting, folding, fixing and dressing hair. Previously these techniques were separated out and students had to learn them as individual disciplines, which made them difficult to grasp. In reality, these skills overlap and often one thing used in dressing is also used in plaiting or twisting. So the different skills are now combined in one chapter and you will have the opportunity to learn them all together.

Preparing for the service

Correctly protect and position clients and yourself

Unless you are using heated rollers or the hair has recently been washed, you will need to shampoo and condition the hair before you start. So, after you have put a clean, fresh gown on the client, place a clean towel around their shoulders before moving them to the basin. Check which products you should be using with the stylist and prepare the hair as described in Chapter 6 Shampoo and condition hair.

When preparing for **wet setting**:

◆ detangle the hair first (remember to work through the point ends first and then work back up the hair to nearer the root)

◆ make sure that the client is comfortable

◆ get the stylist to check that the hair is ready for the service.

When preparing for plaiting and twisting:

◆ detangle the hair first (remember to work through the point ends first and then work back up the hair to nearer the root)

◆ blow-dry the hair into style with a flat brush to keep the hair as smooth as possible

◆ make sure that the client is comfortable

◆ get the stylist to check that the hair is ready for the service.

When you are ready to start, ask the stylist if you should place a plastic cape around the client instead of a towel. Many setting, plaiting and twisting techniques use products like setting lotions or thermal sprays, hair glazes, sprays, gels and waxes. You need to keep both the styling gown and client clean throughout the process, so it may be easier to cover the client's shoulders and clothes at the beginning.

A set on short hair should not take longer than around 25 minutes, plus another 15 minutes dressing out. A full head of scalp plaits or twists takes a lot longer. Therefore, the main health and safety concerns relate to your posture because of the length of time spent plaiting or twisting, and the client will also be sat in the chair for a long time and could become stiff and uncomfortable.

Get things ready

Prepare all of the equipment and products that you need beforehand and put them on your trolley.

◆ For setting – get your rollers, pins and clips ready; make sure that you have enough of the correct roller sizes before you start. If you are using heated rollers, make sure that you have enough of the right sizes heating up as it will be rather embarrassing if you run out halfway through and have to wait for another set of rollers to heat up! Finally, find the brushes and combs that you need and put them close at hand.

TOP TIP

Plaiting and twisting takes a long time, so both you and the client need to be comfortable throughout the service.

◆ For plaiting or twisting – gather together the professional **braiding bands** for plaits and twists, the products that you intend to use, and your combs, brushes and sectioning clips. These should be cleaned, sterilized and made ready for use.

Preparing the client

Although you are styling the client's hair you are doing it under the direct supervision of the stylist. They are ultimately responsible for what you do, and therefore you must follow their instructions.

Only use the styling products that they have asked you to use, and complete the work in the sequence of steps that they give you. For instance, if they have specifically said that they want you to start at the front hairline and to work back from there into the rest of the hair, then that is where you must start.

TOP TIP

You need to prepare your trolley before the client sits down. There is nothing worse than having to leave a client halfway through because you have forgotten something.

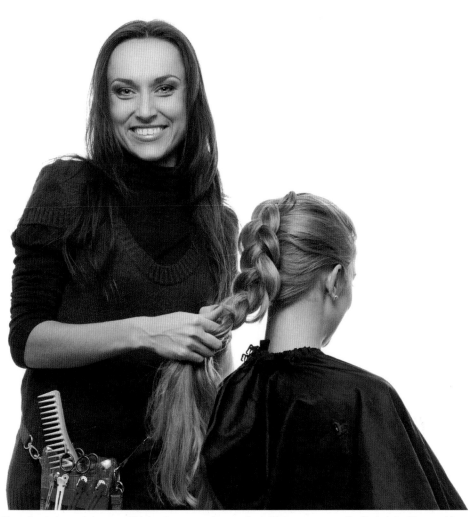

For more information on cleaning, sterilization and general salon hygiene, see Chapter 3 Health and safety.

Dressing hair can be very satisfying for you and your client. Make sure your client's hair is clean and free of tangles, and that your hands are clean and your nails neatly trimmed.

For more information on preparation and maintenance of the salon, tools and equipment, see Chapter 2 Preparing for work.

Preparing for the service (Continued...)

Control your tools

You must work in a controlled way. Carefully divide the hair and secure the areas that you are not yet working on out of the way. Be careful with clips because they can catch on the hair and leave it looking untidy, frizzy or even snap it. Remember, it is impossible to replace untidy lengths of hair once they have been separated from the main stems of hair. Similarly when setting, when the hair has fallen off the edges (shoulders) of the rollers, it will not dry smoothly and will affect the finish of the **comb-out**.

> **TOP TIP**
>
> Never clip hair into a position above the horizontal. This causes the root area to lift and affects the way that the hair will lie after you take it down and want to work with it.

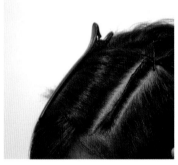

Good sectioning: smooth and flat, with the correct clips

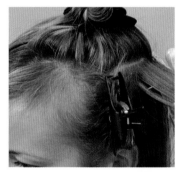

Bad sectioning: hair lifted above the horizontal, the wrong clips used

> **TOP TIP**
>
> When creating scalp plaits and twists you need to apply a styling product whilst you work with the hair. Apply the product after you section the hair and before you position the plait or twist.

> **ACTIVITY**
>
> Any long hair design work needs to be planned from the outset. Choose either a plaiting technique or a twisting technique. Research different effects that can be achieved by using this technique in different ways. Use style magazines and websites to find and gather the information. After collecting together images and sketches of what you would like to do, choose one effect that you would like to re-create. Prepare a practice block by washing, drying, conditioning and detangling the hair. When it is ready, practise the techniques. When you have finished, take photos of the finished effects for your portfolio.

Maintaining personal hygiene standards

Everything that you use must be clean and hygienic; this will prevent the risk of cross-infection and help to maintain a healthy, safe environment. Similarly, your own personal standards of health and hygiene should not present any risk to the client.

For more information on preventing infection and personal health and hygiene, see Chapter 2 Health and safety.

> **TOP TIP**
>
> Flat-jawed clips are easier to work with than 'spiky' crocodile clips. Flat clips will keep the sections of hair that you are not yet working on smooth. They will stop the hair from bulking out and eliminate the problems of crimped hair. Crimped hair is caused by haphazard sectioning and twisting of the hair in a way that it would not normally lie.

Completing the service within an acceptable timescale

Different salons have their own ways of doing things, each with its own appointment scheduling system. Nevertheless, remember that both the client and the stylist have other things to do as well.

If you have problems with the client's hair, stop and get help – do not progress further as it may have a knock-on effect on the whole style and the client may need to be started all over again. Keep an eye on the time so that you do not overrun or make the client late.

The following table provides a rough guideline for how long each type of work will take:

Length	Setting: wet or heated rollers	French plait	Cornrows (10 rows)	Twists (10 scalp twists)	Twists (40 off the head)
shoulder length at one length	25 minutes	20 minutes	1½ hours	1 hour	2–2½ hours
beyond shoulder at one length	30 minutes	25 minutes	2 hours	1½ hours	
short layered length 10–15cm	20 minutes		1½ hours	1½ hours	1½ hours
mid-length layered	25 minutes		1½ hours	1½ hours	2 hours
long layered	30 minutes	25 minutes	2 hours	1½ hours	2 hours

> **TOP TIP**
>
> Plaiting and twisting is intricate work. If your tension on the hair starts to relax, it will be noticeable at the end. You need to pay attention to this and fix it as you go along.

> **TOP TIP**
>
> You need to operate like a professional, so if you are given the responsibility to do the service on a client it must be up to standard.

ACTIVITY

Preparing for plaiting and twisting hair

Copy the table and fill in the missing information.

Preparation	What do you need to do?
Client	
Yourself	
Tools/materials	

> **TOP TIP**
>
> Listen to the stylist: they know the best way to tackle the hair.

Setting and dressing hair

Setting, finishing and heat protection

There is a wide range of products available for you to use; get to know the ones that your salon has. The products that you use will fall into the following categories:

- Setting solutions – mousses and thermal setting sprays protect the hair from excessive heat whilst the hair is being moulded into shape. They are applied to the hair evenly and help the set stay in for longer. Different strengths are used for differing hair types and holds.

- Finishing products enhance the hair by adding shine or gloss, and improve handling and control by removing static, fluffiness or frizz from the hair. Certain finishing products like waxes will define the movement in hair, giving texture or spikiness. Some products laminate the outer cuticle layer, protecting it from the environment. Moroccan Oil™ contains Argan oil.

- Heat protection products provide protection from heat styling. Regular use of straightening irons could damage the hair. A number of products can be applied to reduce any long-term negative effects.

Other products provide protection from harsh UV rays in sunlight in a variety of 'leave-in' treatments that can be used at any time. They are applied before exposure to harsh sunlight and can be washed out. This is particularly useful for clients who have coloured hair, as the bleaching effects of sunlight will quickly remove colour.

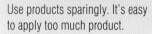

TOP TIP

Use products sparingly. It's easy to apply too much product.

Many of the items you need for setting hair are described in Chapter 2 Preparing for work. Refer to this chapter for more information on rollers, combs, brushes, grips and pins.

Rollering hair

There are various sizes and shapes of roller. When using rollers you need to decide on the size and shape, how you will curl the hair on to them and the position in which you will attach them to the base.

Rules for using rollers:	Common rollering problems:
Small rollers produce tight curls, giving hair more movement.	Rollers not secured properly on base – either dragged or flattened; will not produce lift and volume in the final style.
Large rollers produce loose curls, making hair wavy as opposed to curly.	Too large a hair section – will produce reduced movement in the final result.
On-base rollering produces root lift/volume and end curl.	Too small a hair section – will produce increased movement or curl in the final result.
Off-base rollering produces end curl without root lift.	Longer hair requires larger rollers unless tighter effects are wanted.
The direction in which the hair is wound affects the movement in the final result.	Poorly positioned hair overfalling the sides of the roller will affect the movement in the final result.
	Incorrectly wound hair around the roller will create 'fish hook' ends.
	Twisted hair around the roller will distort the final movement of the style.

STEP-BY-STEP: WET-SET ROLLERING

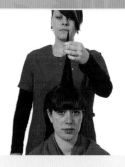

1 Section the hair ready to brick wind the first large curler just behind the client's fringe. Take care to ensure the section is no wider than the roller's footprint.

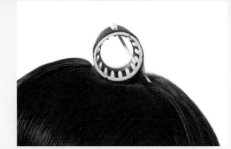

2 Look at the roller from the side view to check that the roots are correctly lifted and the pin inserted at the correct angle.

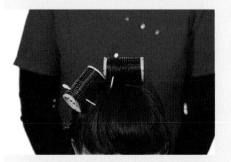

3 Wind another roller to rest adjacent to the first one, and repeat this step.

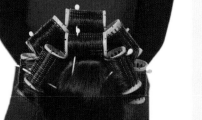

4 Place more rollers to create a brickwork effect ready for the client to sit under the dryer.

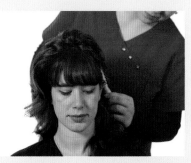

5 When the hair is dry, carefully unwind each roller from the nape upwards, taking care not to stretch the curls. Use a wide-toothed brush and your fingers to shape the hair.

6 The finished effect is long flowing waves.

TOP TIP

Always let the hair cool before removing all the rollers. Hot hair may seem dry when you first check it, but when it cools it may actually be damp.

TOP TIP

If you are not sure which size roller to use, go for the smaller. If necessary you can brush out and stretch hair that is too tightly curled later. Loosely curled hair will drop more readily so you may not achieve the style you were aiming for.

Dressing hair

Dressing is the final styling process of setting. Whereas the setting process provides volume, curls or waves, the dressing-out now blends and smooths these pre-set movements into an overall flowing shape. Dressing uses brushing and combing techniques and dressing aids such as dressing crèmes and hairspray to keep the hair in place. If you have set the hair carefully and accurately, then only the minimum of dressing is required.

Step-by-step: Brushing out

Brushing out the hair blends the waves or curls by removing the partings or set marks created at the curl bases during rollering. It also removes the stiffness caused by setting lotions that aid the hold of the set.

1. One way of achieving the finished dressing is by using a brush and your hand. The thicker the hair, the stiffer the brush bristles need to be. Choose a brush that will flow through the hair comfortably.

2. Apply the brush to the hair ends. Use firm but gentle strokes.

3. Work up the head, starting from the back of the neck.

4. Brush through the waves or curls you have set, gradually moulding the hair into shape.

5. As you brush, pat the hair with your hand to guide the hair into shape. Remember not to over-handle the hair as this can spoil the set.

Back-brushing

Back-brushing is a technique used to give more height and volume to hair. By brushing backwards from the points to the roots you roughen the cuticle of the hair. The hair will now tangle slightly and bind together to hold a fuller shape. The amount of hair back-brushed determines the fullness of the finished style. Most textures of hair can be back-brushed. It adds bulk and makes the hair easier to manage. The technique is especially useful with fine hair.

Step-by-step: Back-brushing

1. Hold a section of hair out from the head; for maximum life, hold the section straight out from the head and apply the back-brushing close to the roots.

2. Place the brush at the top of the held section at an angle slightly dipping in to the held section of hair.

3. Now, with a slight turn outwards with the wrist, turn and push down a small amount of hair towards the scalp.

4. Repeat this in a few adjacent sections of hair.

5. Smooth out the longer lengths in the direction required, covering the tangled back-brushed hair beneath.

TOP TIP

Back-combing is applied to the underside of the hair section. Do not let the comb penetrate too deeply, otherwise the final dressing and smoothing out will remove the support you have put in.

Alternatively, use back-combing. This technique is similar to back-brushing except that a comb is used rather than a brush to turn back the shorter hairs within a section. This provides firmer support and volume than back-brushing, as back-combing is applied deeper toward the scalp. It provides a stronger, longer lasting result. Back-brushing is harder to remove and is more damaging to the hair

Use the workstation mirror

As you work, keep using the mirror to check the shape that you are creating. If you find the outer style-line is misshapen or lacking volume, do not be afraid to go back to re-section and back-brush/comb again. When you have finished the look, hold a back mirror at an angle to maximize what the client can see of their hairstyle.

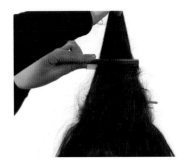

Back-combing is an alternative to back-brushing

STEP-BY-STEP: HEATED ROLLER SET

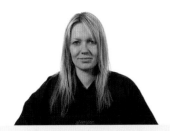

1 Prepare your client with a clean fresh gown.

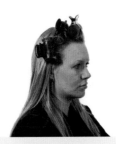

2 Start by placing the rollers into the hair, starting at the front.

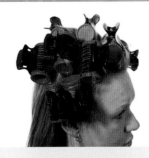

3 As you progress through the set, check with the client that the rollers are not too hot. You can use pieces of neck wool to cushion each roller at the scalp.

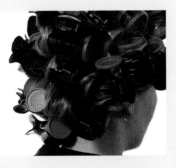

4 Leave the rollers in until they have all cooled down.

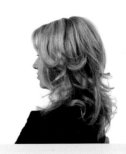

5 Carefully remove the rollers, starting at the bottom (not at the top) of the head.

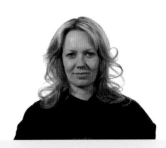

6 Work through the hair with your fingers, without brushing, to create this loosely dressed effect.

Plaiting and twisting hair

Securing the free ends of plaits

As cornrows and scalp twists extend beyond the contour of the head, the freely hanging lengths need to be secured to create a finish:

◆ nearer to the head by sewing with thread using a curved needle or by using professional bands to allow the remainder of the hair to be styled in some other way

◆ nearer the ends of the plait or twist using professional bands. This enables the freely hanging plaits/twists to create an overall braided effect.

Learning about hair textures

Certain hair textures suit specific styling. For example, a head of cornrows on African Caribbean hair is probably better finished in free hanging plaits rather than with heat styling. Alternatively, European hair may be slippery and will need to be well secured.

> **TOP TIP**
>
> Plaiting and twisting is a step-by-step procedure. If you miss one out it will impact on the rest of the style.

> **TOP TIP**
>
> Always use professional bands – these will be less damaging to the client's hair than using any other type of elastic or rubber band.

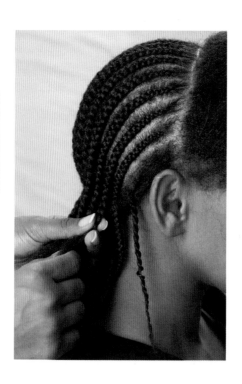

> **TOP TIP**
>
> Always detangle the hair and brush it through as you work through each section or stem of hair.

Straight hair is easier to style in plaits rather than twists, whereas curly hair can be cornrowed or twisted. Freely hanging ends of scalp plaits or twists can be crimped, waved or curled.

Maintaining an even tension

The stylist will provide you with the necessary instructions because they know the best way of completing the work to achieve a satisfactory result. Be careful with your tensioning as you handle and manipulate the hair. Obviously you do not want to hurt the client or damage their hair, but you do need to maintain an even pressure so that the hair lies properly in the design. If hair starts to 'bulk out' within a plait while you are working on it, unravel it and do the plait again – it will not get any better the longer you leave it, it actually gets worse.

If a client says the plait or twist is pulling and painful you will have to ease the stress on the root of the hair that is pulling at the scalp. First find the area that is the problem. This may show as tension and lifting at the scalp. Then decide whether the end of a tail comb can ease and loosen the stem of hair, or whether you have to undo and start that plait again.

Sort the problems out as you go   When you encounter problems with the technique that you are trying to apply, stop. Get your stylist to help or give you some advice on how to tackle the problem. A lot of plaiting and twisting work is sequential. This means that you need to do A before B and B before C etc. If something goes wrong at B and you do not sort it out there and then, and just carry on to finish, you may not be able to correct it very easily. So make sure each step is correct before moving on to the next step.

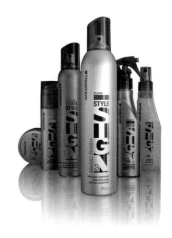

Applying suitable products

The products that you will be using will do one of the following:

- provide hold, while you work, by bonding the hair together
- finish the hair, improving the look and feel
- provide a final hold, bonding the finished hairstyle in place.

Quite simply, a hairstyle that is designed to last for a longer time, such as scalp plaits, scalp twists and off-the-head twists, needs something to fix it in position or give it hold.

There are two main forms of hair product:

- Styling products such as gels and pomades contain fixatives to hold and support the hair in its shape whilst you are handling the hair, giving it definition and shape.
- Finishing products include serums and sprays, which add shine and lustre to improve the look of the hair or provide a final fix.

The choice of what you use should be made by the stylist, as they will know what effect they are trying to achieve and what will work best with the hair. Products like wax, serum or gel come in what seems like relatively small containers. This is because these products are highly concentrated and a very small amount goes a long way.

TOP TIP

Always use styling and finishing products sparingly because it is easy to overload the hair – if you do, it may need to be re-washed and the styling re-started! It is also poor economy, as these products are expensive and it is a waste of the salon's resources.

TOP TIP

Always follow the manufacturer's instructions when using any styling or finishing products.

TOP TIP

Plaits are free-hanging stem(s) of hair that show off hair length. This length can be natural or can be extended by adding hair during the plaiting process; an example is the French or **fishtail plait**.

Plaiting and twisting hair (Continued...)

Styling products

Product	Suitability	Purpose	Application	If over-applied
Dry wax	suitable for bonding the ends of cornrows and twists	moderately firm hold providing a non-wet look or greasy finish	applied in small amounts with the fingertips into ends of the hair	easy to add too much and overload the hair, particularly on finer hair types
Normal (grease-based) wax	suitable for bonding the lengths and ends of cornrows and twists	firm hold; high definition and texture with a moist or slightly wet look effect	applied in small amounts with the fingertips into lengths of the hair during the initial separation of strands	easy to add too much and overload the hair, particularly on finer hair types
Hair gel	suitable for bonding the lengths and ends of cornrows and twists	wet look effect with very strong hold when gel dries into position	applied with fingertips or comb; it is easy to see where it has been missed	you can't overload the hair as the look is based on 100% coverage
Styling glaze	suitable for bonding the lengths and ends of cornrows	wet look effect with firm-strong hold when it dries into position	applied first to the hands and rubbed into the hair all over; plait the hair; apply more if it dries	you can't overload the hair as the look is based on 100% coverage
Serum	suitable for **French plaits**	improves handling, provides shine; smooths out frizzes while plaiting	applied in small amounts with the finger tips into pre-plaited hair	it is easy to overload the hair, making it greasy
Fixing sprays – mild, moderate and firm hold	plaits and twists	used as a final fixative or as a styling product if scrunched into 'fanned' ends	applied to pre-dried hair by directional spraying from 30cm away	too much will make hair 'crunchy'

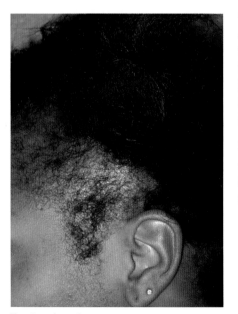

Traction alopecia

Traction alopecia

One of the more serious after-effects of wearing hair in any scalp-plaited or scalp-twisted hairstyle is **traction alopecia**. This occurs when constant pressure is applied to the roots of the hair. This can result in hair loss in patches on the scalp, showing as baldness, and is particularly obvious in areas of weaker hair such as the temples or hairlines.

If the client tells you that they have an unpleasant tightness in any area as you are working, try releasing the pressure by using the pointed end of a tail comb to ease the stems of the plaits. If this does not release the tension, you will have to remove the plait or twist and re-start that area again.

Creating plaits and twists

Plaiting is a method of intertwining three or more strands of hair to create a variety of woven hairstyles. When done for specific occasions it is often decorated by ornamentation, such as fresh flowers, glass or plastic beads. Coloured silks and added hair are also popular. The final effect is dependent upon:

◆ the number of plaits or twists used

◆ the positioning of the plait or twist across the scalp or around the head

◆ the way in which the plaits are made (under or over)

◆ the addition of ornamentation/decoration or added hair applied.

TOP TIP

If there is an imbalance in the tension of the strands while you plait, see if you can even it out by carefully lifting the tightest strands with the end of a tail comb.

CourseMate video: Basic plait

STEP-BY-STEP: LOOSE PLAITING (THREE-STEM LOOSE PLAIT)

The three-stem plait is easily achieved and demonstrates the basic principle of plaiting hair.

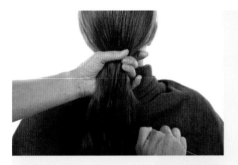

1 Brush and comb the hair thoroughly before starting. You may find it useful to keep the hair slightly damp.

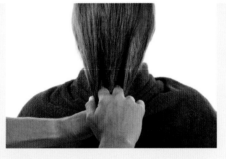

2 Hold the hair with one hand, using the fingers of your free hand to separate the hair into three sections.

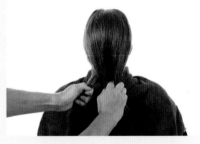

3 Hold the sections tightly and place one of the side sections over the centre one. Repeat this technique using the section from the other side of the centre one.

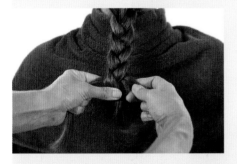

4 Continue placing the outside sections of hair over the centre ones until you reach the ends of the stems.

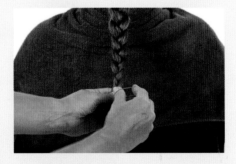

5 Secure the free ends with thread or a professional band.

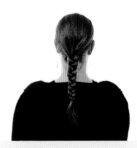

6 Once you can achieve this plait well other plaits will be easier to master.

Plaiting and twisting hair (Continued...)

French plait   The French plait is a simple but attractive way of wearing longer hair down, secured, but not loose. In hairdressing terms, it falls into what we call hair-ups. Many clients tend to have French plaits for specific occasions such as weddings, parties and formal evenings out. Clients with long hair (and hair extensions) can display the length of their hair whilst having it controlled; it is often finished off with a themed decoration with some form of hair ornament.

Cornrow   The cornrow is a type of three-stem plait. However, it is secured closer to the scalp to create head-hugging patterned designs that can last up to four weeks.

Cornrows (also known as cane rows) originated in Africa and have been a unique way of displaying hair art and design, often incorporating complex patterns indicating status or tribal connection. In fact, as this art form has been passed down for thousands of years it is quite probable that the very first hairdressers worked on these elaborate techniques.

Cornrows create design patterns across the scalp by working along predefined channels of hair. These channels are secured to the scalp by interlocking each of the three subdivided stems as the plaiting technique progresses. Short or even layered hair can be made to look longer if extension hair is added during the process. The added hair is plaited into the style along each of the sections that create the plaited effect.

Cornrows have become a popular way of wearing finely detailed scalp plaits that can form straight, curved or zigzag patterns, swirls, circles and wavy designs. The techniques were originally produced by African tribes to define their identities, but have become a popular option for any hair type. Good cornrowing is intricate, attractive, highly detailed and long lasting, and the technique is quickly becoming a modern classic.

TOP TIP

The tension used in plaiting can exert exceptional pressure on the hair follicle. Scalp-type plaits or cornrows are more vulnerable than free-hanging plaits. In extreme cases this may cause hair loss; areas of hair become thin and baldness may even result! Traction alopecia is particularly obvious at the temples of younger girls with long hair who regularly wear their hair tied up for school, sport or dancing.

TOP TIP

When cornrows have been applied to the hair, the effect can last up to six weeks or more before they should be removed. Advice should be given on handling and maintaining the hair, although regular shampooing can still be carefully achieved.

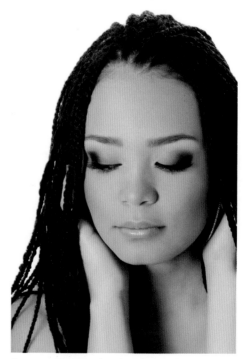

Cornrows involve a lot of work and take a lot of time with beautiful results

STEP-BY-STEP: THREE-STEM FRENCH PLAITING

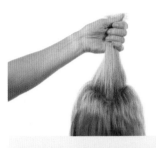

1 Section the hair at the front hairline into a triangle. Divide this section into three equal strands as if you were starting a basic plait.

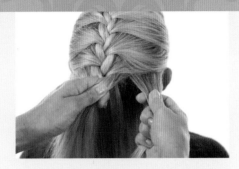

2 Hold one of the strands in one hand and two of the strands in the other. Add a little extra hair from the front hairline into the outer strand.

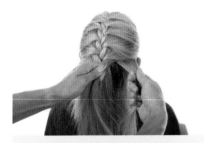

3 Pass the outer strand and extra hair across and into the centre and into your other hand.

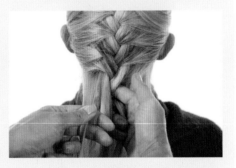

4 Do the same on the other side and repeat this technique all the way down the hair.

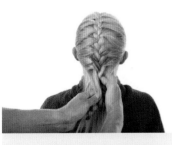

5 Continue steps 3 and 4 taking in a new section of hair from the hairline each time.

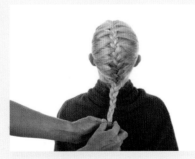

6 Your French plait will now start to form. Continue the plait in the same way until you finish.

TOP TIP

Hair products designed especially for these services are often very different from the everyday styling products you would use in other styling services. Use these products in line with manufacturer's instructions and be careful not to overload the hair during the styling process. Once the product has been applied to the hair it will be difficult to remove it without re-washing.

TOP TIP

Regardless of whether you are doing scalp plaits, singles or twists, the direction in which they flow is related to their starting position on the scalp. Your accurate sectioning creates this.

CourseMate video: French plait

CourseMate video: Cornrowing

Plaiting and twisting hair (Continued...)

STEP-BY-STEP: CORNROWING

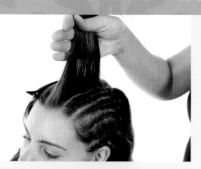

1 Decide on the linear design you want to create first, as this will have an impact on where you start. Section off a channel of hair that is the length of the scalp plait required.

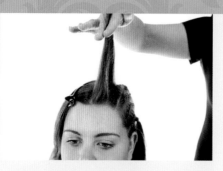

2 Section all the other hair out of the way with flat clips.

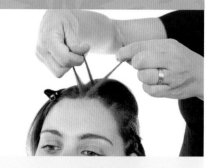

3 Take a small section from the front and divide it into three stems.

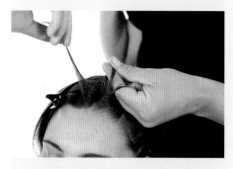

4 Cross over the left and right stems, under the central one.

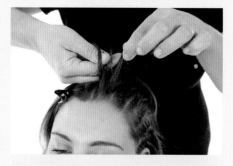

5 To progress along the scalp, pick up a small section and incorporate it into the left stem and move the left stem over the central stem. Now repeat on the right side.

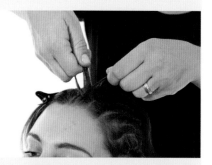

6 Repeat Step 5 until you have worked along the scalp to the desired point.

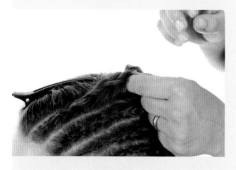

7 Remember to keep the plait taut with an even tension to avoid 'bagging'.

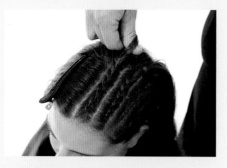

8 When you have reached the end of the plait, secure the remainder with a braiding band.

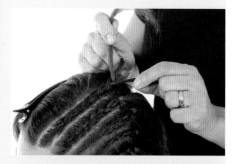

9 Complete the other cornrows using the same technique.

STEP-BY-STEP: FISHTAIL PLAITS

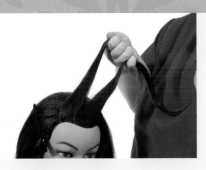

1 A fishtail plait differs from other plaiting techniques as it involves four stems rather than three. Start by separating the hair into two stems.

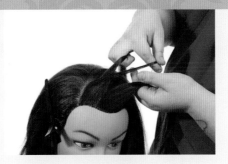

2 While holding each stem in each hand, sub-divide each one, taking the outer narrower stem and passing it across the other and into the centre

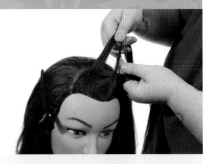

3 Do the same with the other side – sub-divide and pass the outer stem over and into the centre.

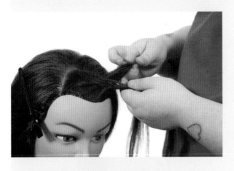

4 Repeat this movement and work down the hair length.

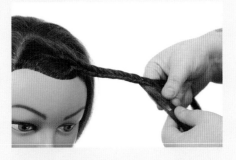

5 The front fishtail is now clearly formed.

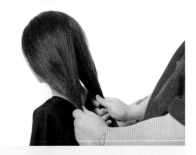

6 Now repeat the same sequence of movements at the back of the hair, from the crown.

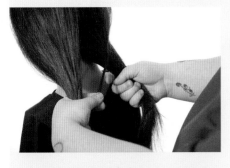

7 While holding each stem in each hand, sub-divide each one, taking the outer narrower stem and passing it across the other and in the centre.

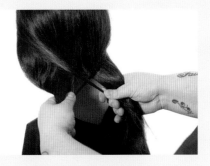

8 Repeat this process with the other side, sub-dividing the hair stems and passing the outer over and into the centre.

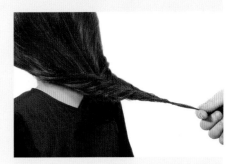

9 Repeat this movement and work down to the ends of the hair to give the unique fishtail look.

Plaiting and twisting hair (Continued...)

Twists are an alternative to plaited styles, but unlike plaits, they do not involve any interlocking of hair. Twists produce a lovely thick rope-like braid which makes a change from a plait. It is best suited to medium long or long hair.

STEP-BY-STEP: ROPE PLAIT OR TWIST

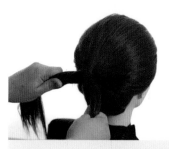

1 Fix the hair centrally at the back in a pony with a covered band. Then divide the pony into two equal sections.

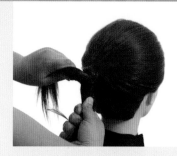

2 Now twist both stems in a clockwise direction.

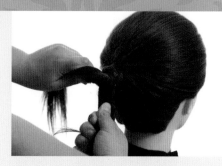

3 Wind the twisted stems around each other.

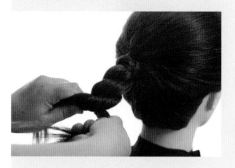

4 Using a firm grip, twist and wind the length of the stems.

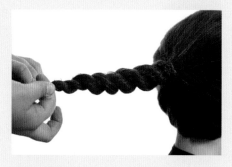

5 Continue this pattern until a rope-like effect is achieved.

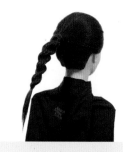

6 Use a braiding band to bond the ends together for the finished effect.

TOP TIP

If hair is left in a plaited or twisted style for too long, the quality and condition of the hair can deteriorate. Potential effects include:

- dryness and brittleness – the hair lacks moisture

- hair damage or breakage

- traction alopecia from constant root tension

- knotted or matted hair, which is impossible to remove without cutting

- scalp dryness and flaking.

SUMMARY

Now you have finished this chapter you should have a clearer picture of all the essential aspects associated with dressing, plaiting and twisting hair. In particular, you should now have a good understanding and be able to:

✓ prepare the clients for dressing, plaiting and twisting services

✓ describe the detrimental effects that plaiting and twisting can have if done incorrectly

✓ know when to use and apply setting and dressing products during the service

✓ carry out basic setting, dressing, plaiting and twisting techniques using a variety of different tools and equipment.

In addition, you will understand how these processes will enable you to work more efficiently and effectively in daily salon routines.

REVISION QUESTIONS

Q1. Copy and complete this sentence: _____ alopecia is a condition caused by excessive tension upon the hair.   Fill in the blank

Q2. A 'rope plait' is an effect created by twisting the hair?   True or False

Q3. Which of the following techniques would take less than 30 minutes to complete? (You may choose more than one answer.)

a French plait	☐	a
a full head of cornrows	☐	b
a 'pony' tail	☐	c
a full head of scalp twists	☐	d
a full head of cane rows	☐	e
a full head of twisted knots	☐	f

Q4. Cornrows are a close 'head hugging' design made up of several scalp plaits?   True or False

Q5. Which of the following is the odd one out? (Choose one answer.)

cornrows	○	a
fishtail plait	○	b
rope plait	○	c
French plait	○	d

9 Assist with Removing Hair Extensions

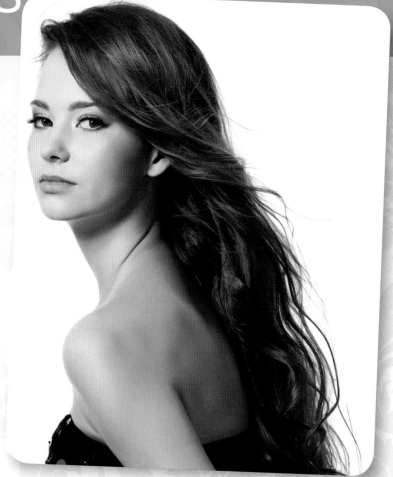

LEARNING OBJECTIVES

When you have finished this chapter you should:

◆ be able to work safely and carefully when removing hair extensions

◆ be able to remove a variety of hair extension systems

◆ know how wearing hair extensions can affect hair

◆ know your salon's policies and legal obligations

◆ know how to communicate professionally with clients.

KEY TERMS

avant-garde

cold-fusion hair extensions

hair additions

hair alternatives

hair enhancements

hot-bonded hair extensions

maintenance appointments

plaited and braided extensions

removal solution

removal tool

sewn-in extensions

INFORMATION COVERED IN THIS CHAPTER

PRACTICAL SKILLS

Learn to work carefully and safely when assisting with hair extension services

Learn how to work with and remove a variety of hair extensions

Learn how to work with a variety of real and synthetic hair extension systems

Learn how to work with a range of hair extension tools and equipment

UNDERPINNING KNOWLEDGE

Know salon and legal requirements

Understand the problems that can arise from wearing hair extensions

Know how to use the tools and equipment associated with hair extension services

Know how to communicate effectively and professionally

Know how to use hair extension removal techniques

INTRODUCTION

Hair extensions have been a popular accessory for several decades. At first, the contemporary hair extension service was a very exclusive one, and with a price tag to match. Like many other fashions that start on catwalks across the world, the exclusivity factor becomes appealing to the mass market as well. Ultimately, technology and mass production processes step in and manufacturers find ways to make this service something that anyone can afford.

There are many types of hair extension systems available today and several ways to attach them to hair. Wearing them is one thing, but they do not last forever as they need maintenance and removal at some point. This chapter shows you the variety of extension systems available and how you can contribute to the service and its maintenance.

Different hair extension systems and styles

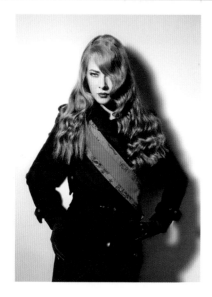

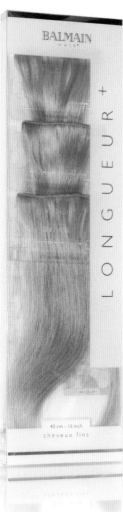

There are four main systems for applying strands or wefts of extension hair into a client's hairstyle:

◆ hot-bonded

◆ cold-fusion

◆ plaited/braided

◆ sewn-in.

Each of these systems has a particular method for removal, and you will need to be familiar with all the techniques.

Hot-bonded extension system
This is a popular and widely used hair extension system for longer lasting effects. Heated tools are used to melt a polymer resin, creating a hard bond that attaches the extensions near the root area of the client's natural hair. It is suitable for all hair types except African Caribbean hair and allows the stylist to apply individual extension strands to create freely flowing hairstyles that move like real hair. This system uses a removal tool (similar to a pair of pliers) to break the seals and remove the extension from the hair. The hair can then be prepared for further services.

Cold-fusion extension system
This type of system uses adhesives, solutions or tapes to hold strands or wefts of extension hair in place on natural hair. Cold-fusion systems create bonds that can be used on any hair type. Regardless of the method used, they are removed by the careful application of a chemical bond-removing solution.

Plaited/braided extensions
This method uses plaiting techniques to add extension hair into a hairstyle. This does not produce a freely flowing hairstyle but can be applied to many hair lengths and types. These are removed by carefully cutting them out of the client's natural hair.

Sewn-in extensions
This is a popular system for applying wefts of natural or synthetic fibre extensions on to pre-plaited scalp braids called cornrows. The wefts are sewn onto the braids using a curved needle and thread. They are particularly popular on African Caribbean hair and other curly hair types. Removal involves great care as, like plaits and braids, they are cut to release them from the client's natural hair.

Hair extension hairstyles

Four types of effect can be created by hair extensions:

◆ hair additions

◆ hair extensions

◆ hair enhancements

◆ hair alternatives.

Hair additions are applied as strands to give subtle or vibrant contrasts to the client's own colour, for example as highlights, lowlights, colour flashes and slices. This system provides an alternative to permanent colouring and adds more fibre or hair to the client's original hair, making the hair thicker than before. This is particularly useful if the client has fine hair.

Hair enhancements can be applied as strands but more popularly as rows of wefts. They will thicken the client's natural hair, giving more body, and make the natural hair look longer. They are quick to apply, available in a wide range of natural and synthetic hair colours and lengths, and reusable if they are looked after and maintained.

Hair extensions are applied using 150–250 individual strand extensions that can be either pre-bonded natural hair or synthetic fibre. The colours can be matched to the client's own hair, giving natural effects, can be multi-toned as highlights or lowlights, or blended to give a variety of fashion effects. These give clients an immediate, longer, free-flowing hairstyle.

Hair alternatives are a textured fibre or real hair extension made by the stylist into a braid, a twisted effect like a dreadlock, or any unnaturally occurring effect. These styles are more **avant-garde** in their appearance.

> **TOP TIP**
>
> After three months the remaining original extensions will be so far away from the scalp that they must all be removed, even if only to be replaced with new hair extensions.

Maintenance

Hair extensions do not last forever. Even if they are applied to the root area using a hot-bonded system they will gradually grow out. Hair grows at an average rate of 12.5mm per month, so within a couple of months the extensions could be more than 25mm (2.5cm) away from the scalp. Nevertheless, because of general wear and tear, many of these will need replacing to tidy up. **Maintenance appointments** for hair extensions are an essential part of the complete service. When the hair extension specialist initially consults with the client, they will be looking for an ongoing commitment in maintaining the look. This means that the client will book their tidy-up appointment around four to six weeks after the original extension service. During this appointment the hair extension specialist will select the extensions that need to be replaced. You will be removing these so that the hair is prepared for the re-application of new extensions in this area.

The complete head of extensions needs to be removed during the removal appointment so that the hair can be reconditioned and made ready for further extensions or other services. The removal appointment is the final hair extension maintenance appointment, which is booked 12 weeks after the original hair extensions were applied.

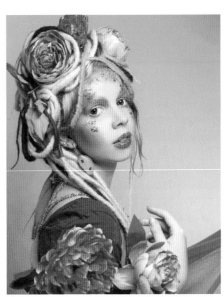

Hair alternatives can be bold and avant-garde

The length of time booked for the removal of extensions during the maintenance appointment will depend on the bonding system used. For example, a full head of extensions applied by a hot-bonded system can take up to three hours. A partial head replacement of extensions for the same system can take up to an hour or so to remove. However, the removal of sewn-in extensions may take considerably less time because complete wefts of hair are quicker to remove than strands. When the thread is cut the whole weft is released, leaving the natural hair in its braided scalp plaits effect.

> **TOP TIP**
>
> We naturally lose 80 to 100 hairs per day. These are normally replaced at the same rate with new hair so we do not end up prematurely bald. However, for clients with hair extensions, this hair fall creates another problem. As the hair grows and falls away from the scalp, it cannot fall away from the hairstyle because it is bonded to the extensions. Within three months this looks very fluffy or fuzzy because the entwined hair will tangle and the frizziness can't be combed away. Some bonds can leave tiny knots in the natural hair around the root area that can be very difficult to comb out.

Working safely while providing services to clients

ACTIVITY

Preparing for hair extension removal

Copy the table and fill in the missing information.

Preparation	What do you need to do?
Client	
Yourself	
Tools/materials	

Correctly protect and position clients and yourself

Make sure that the client is adequately protected throughout the service. They should be wearing a full gown and towel, and possibly a cape too, so that they are protected from falling hair clippings, hard sealant fragments and spills from **removal solutions**.

A full head of hair extensions – even temporary ones – takes a long time to apply and removal time can be equally long. Therefore, the main health and safety concerns relate to the length of time that you will be standing while doing the work, and the client's comfort, positioning and protection during the process.

In addition to your posture and positioning, you must take every care in the way that you handle and use the equipment because:

- it is easy to spill removal chemicals on the client
- you may be using removal equipment that could easily slip and injure you or the client, or damage their hair
- you will need to keep an even tension on the client's hair while you work, without putting too much pressure on their hair or scalp.

Keeping work areas clean at all times

The work area must be clean – workstations, hairdressing trolleys, any work surfaces and surrounding floor areas must be kept spotless. Keep cotton wool swabs and cloths close at hand so that you can quickly attend to any chemical spills on the client or the floor.

Maintaining personal hygiene standards

All the materials that come into contact with the client's skin must be clean and hygienic. Similarly, your own personal standards of health and hygiene should not present any risk to the client. This will prevent the risk of cross-infection and helps to maintain a healthy, safe environment.

TOP TIP

The removal of hair extensions takes a long time. This is true even for a tidy-up appointment, and you will be standing throughout the process. Take particular care with your standing position and your posture to avoid fatigue.

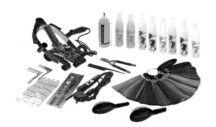

Risks associated with hair extension services

There are some specific risks associated with hair extension services. These are outlined below.

You must	...because there is a risk that
Keep your nails trimmed, and hands and jewellery clean	... you might pass on infections with dirty hands, nails or jewellery.
Keep jewellery on your hands or around your wrists to a minimum	... if jewellery gets caught in the extensions they may need cutting out to remove them.
Wear comfortable, loose-fitting clothes and shoes	... you will tire and feel uncomfortable very quickly as you will be standing for a long period.
Make sure that your client is sitting in a height-adjustable chair	... you will get back ache, neck ache or fatigue if you work in the wrong position.
Sterilize the tools that you will be using on the client	... you could cross-infect the client by using unhygienic tools.
Work in a well-ventilated area when you use removal solutions	... you or the client could become ill from the vapours these products give off.
Clear up any chemical spills immediately	... the floor will become slippery and a hazard to everyone. ... if these spill on to the client it could damage their clothes.
Wear disposable vinyl gloves when handling removal solutions	... these products could cause contact dermatitis – see Chapter 3 for more information.

For more information on preventing infection and personal health and hygiene, see Chapter 3 Health and safety.

TOP TIP

Always wear the PPE (disposable gloves and plastic apron) provided by your salon when carrying out technical services.

ACTIVITY

Copy the table below. For each of the things listed, write down the safety considerations associated with it and what you should do to avoid hazards or risks.

Area of work	Safety consideration	What should you do to avoid hazards or risks?
Cold-fusion systems		
Hot-bonded systems		
Standing during the removal process		
Keeping the work area tidy		

Using tools and materials safely

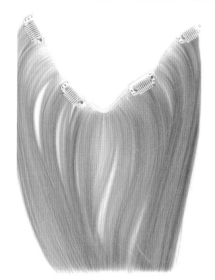

A synthetic fibre extension weft

You will be handling and using many of the tools and materials that the hair extension specialists use in their work, so you must be familiar with how they are used safely and correctly.

Synthetic (artificial) fibre extension hair

Synthetic or artificial extension hair is a man-made fibre that is specifically designed to create hair extension hairstyles. It is pre-coloured in a wide range of tones and is prepared to provide the following textures:

- straight lengths in strands or wefts
- ringlets as wefts
- wavy lengths as wefts
- plaits as wefts
- curly lengths as wefts
- dreadlocks as wefts.

Artificial hair can feel, look and move like natural hair in great condition. It is made from acrylic, which is particularly sensitive to heat. It is very easily damaged or distorted if the fibre is brought into contact with heat or heated equipment. You must take care when handling this material so that you do not affect the quality of the fibre. The hair extension specialist would also have taken a lot of care in handling the fibres when they were first applied. The extension wefts would have been kept flat and smooth so that they did not tangle or knot before they were applied. You should take care when handling the material to avoid tangling and knotting too.

Real extension hair

Real hair extensions are Asian or European in origin. They have been prepared by cleansing in caustic soda (which removes any infestation) and then coloured, lightened or permed to create the required structure. During this processing, the lengths of hair have to be kept in the same root-to-point direction, as shown in the diagram. This has to be followed through during application as well, otherwise the hair will matt or lock together. This occurs because if the hair's natural cuticle layers lie in different directions, the hair tangles and becomes impossible to maintain. Real hair can be bonded together as sewn wefts, bulk lengths or pre-bonded lengths. The weft looks like a curtain of hair. It can be made up into narrow or wide lengths, with the root end being bonded by machine or hand stitching. Take care when handling the material to avoid tangling, as tangled hair cannot be used and is wasteful.

TOP TIP

Hair extensions are pre-processed to create different structures. This refers to the physical appearance of the hair extensions, which can be strands, ringlets, plaits or dreadlocks.

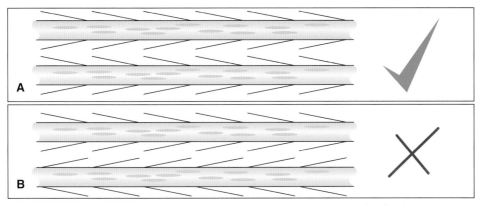

Hair lying with (A) cuticle edges in same direction and (B) cuticle edges in opposite directions

> **TOP TIP**
>
> Real hair extensions must always lie with natural hair in the same root-to-point direction to avoid tangling and matting.

Removal solutions

These chemical products are formulated to work with cold-fusion systems and are applied directly to the bonds to dissolve the adhesive and release the hair extension from the client's natural hair. They are acetone- or alcohol-based and must always be used following the manufacturer's instructions. They are patented products that are matched to specific cold-fusion systems; it is essential that the correct removal solution be used.

Removal tools

Removal tools are metal instruments that look like pliers. They are designed to crush the adhesive bond that holds the extension in place for hot-bonded systems. You must take care when using them because it is very easy to pull or damage the client's hair while removing their extensions. They can be sterilized in the same way that other metal tools are cleaned and maintained in an autoclave or UV cabinet.

For more details on cleaning and maintaining metal tools see the section on sterilization in Chapter 2 Prepare for work.

ACTIVITY

Consider some of the health and safety advice covered so far. Write the answers to the following questions in your portfolio.

1. Why is it important to keep the work area clean and tidy?
2. How is the risk of cross-infection minimized?
3. How should you stand when removing hair extensions?
4. When should you wear PPE and why?
5. How would you know if a client is comfortable or not?

Removing hair extensions

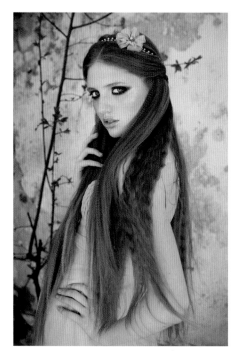

Listen to the hair extension specialist's instructions

The hair extension specialist will have consulted the client and decided on the correct course of action. This will be either:

◆ the removal of selected hair extensions that have grown away from the root area and now need replacing; or

◆ the removal of all the extensions so that the hair is prepared for further services.

You will be working under the close supervision of the specialist; you must follow their instructions.

Minimize the risk of hair damage

Traction alopecia   One of the more serious after effects of wearing hair extensions is traction alopecia. This occurs when a constant pressure, such as wearing hair tied up or weight from hair extensions, is applied to the roots of the hair. It can result in hair loss in patches upon the scalp (baldness), and is particularly obvious in areas of weaker hair such as the temples or hairlines.

If the client tells you that they have had unpleasant tightness in any area since the extensions were applied, you should tell the hair extension specialist immediately because this may affect the removal process. Similarly, if you find sore or thinning areas on the scalp, tell the specialist immediately.

ACTIVITY

Write down your answers to the following questions in your portfolio.

1. What are the signs of traction alopecia?
2. What is the average rate of growth of hair?
3. Why shouldn't a client wear hair extensions for more than three months?
4. What is the difference between a cold-fusion system and a hot-bonded system?
5. What is the difference between a hair addition and a hair alternative?
6. Which way should natural hair extensions lay in relation to a client's own hair?

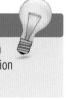

TOP TIP

If you are not sure what has been asked of you, ask the hair extension specialist to explain again.

Ensure that the client is comfortable

Removing extensions takes a long time, even for a tidy-up appointment, and the client will be seated in the same position throughout. Stop now and again to give both you and the client a bit of a break. You could always offer to make them a drink, bring a selection of magazines or suggest that they take a comfort break.

It is often difficult to hold a conversation while you are concentrating on what you are doing. (Do not worry – many experienced stylists have the same problem.) However, long periods of silence can be uncomfortable, particularly when the client does not understand what is going on. Try to be reassuring. People tend to get edgy when they wait for a long time and very little (as far as they are concerned) seems to be happening. Make a point of explaining what you are doing now and then. This keeps them informed and prevents their boredom turning into panic.

The client will sense your level of confidence. If you show signs of anxiety the client will be stressed too. If they then start to panic, you will naturally sense it too and it winds up the stress level. Keep calm; if you find that a particular area or bond is difficult to remove take your time. It will work eventually (you can always call the hair extension specialist for help).

TOP TIP

Taking a pair of pliers to someone's hair can look rather alarming! Explain what you are doing, why you are doing it and roughly how long it will take.

ACTIVITY

This activity considers how the client might be feeling throughout the removal process. Copy the table below into your portfolio and fill in your answers for each of the situations.

Situation	What signs would they be showing?	What would you do?
The client feels anxious about what you are doing		
The client is worried about their hair extensions		
The client is feeling uncomfortable		

TOP TIP

Simple words of reassurance reduce panic and remove stress. Keep things light-hearted – humour is a great way to break down barriers. Reassurance can run along the lines of saying things like: 'Yes, this is normal. It often takes a bit longer to get Steve's extensions out; he puts them in so well.'

TOP TIP

Always check that you are using the correct removal solution for the right cold-fusion system.

Removing hair extensions (Continued...)

Preparing the hair for the service

If the stylist is going to reapply the hair extensions on the same day as the removal, you will need to shampoo the natural hair with a clarifying shampoo prior to the reapplication. This will remove any traces of conditioner or product build-up, which may affect the effectiveness of the bonding of the newly applied extensions. Dry the hair into style and brush well to remove any loose hairs.

> See Chapter 6 for more information on shampooing and conditioning hair.

Learning about removal techniques

Be organized; gather the things that you need on your trolley:

- the correct removal solution
- an old pair of hairdressing scissors
- cotton wool pads
- hair clips
- disposable vinyl gloves
- comb and soft bristle brush
- removal tool.

TOP TIP

Always detangle the hair and brush it through after you remove each hair extension.

Cold-fusion adhesive tape strip removal Self-adhesive extensions need a special chemical spray or solution to dissolve the bond attaching them to the hair, so put on your gloves and apron before doing anything. When the removal solution is applied or sprayed onto the self-cling tape strip, it quickly reduces the adhesion and therefore releases the weft from the hair. The removed weft can then be inspected to see if it is worth keeping or whether it should be thrown away.

The self-cling strips can be removed from the weft in the same way that the extension is removed from the hair. Depending on the quality of the weft, it can be washed, reconditioned and retained for future use, or otherwise disposed of. If the weft is to be reused, new, double-sided self-adhesive tape strips will need to be applied after the wefts have been dried.

Sewn weft removal Using old hairdressing scissors, carefully cut the stitches that hold the weft in place, as shown in the photo to the left. The weft will fall from the natural hair.

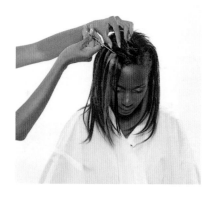

STEP-BY-STEP: HOT-BOND STRAND REMOVAL

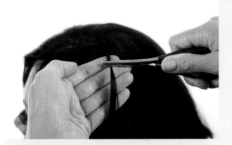

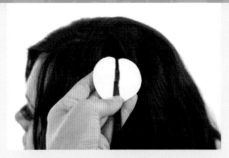

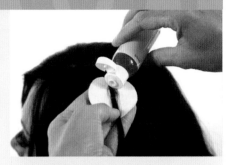

1 Take a removal tool and crush along the length of the bond.

2 Place a cotton wool pad underneath the bond to catch any drips of solution.

3 Apply a removal solution to the bond. Fold the cotton wool pad over the bond and hold it for one to three minutes.

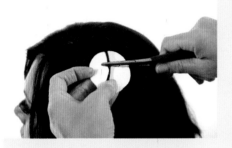

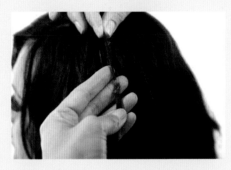

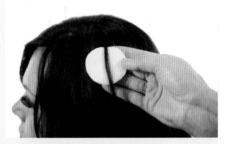

4 Once the solution has penetrated the bond, crush the bond using the removal tool.

5 As the bond crumbles and breaks down, pull the extension hair gently away from the natural hair.

6 The hair extension is removed.

CourseMate video: Removing hair extensions (cold fusion)

Removing hair extensions (Continued...)

STEP-BY-STEP: COLD-FUSION BONDED WEFT REMOVAL

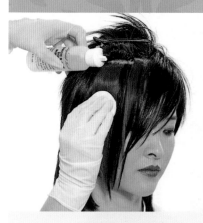

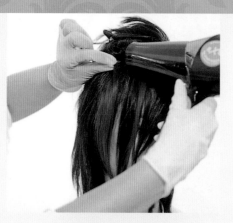

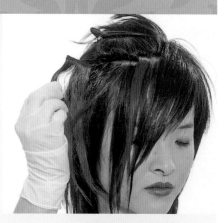

1 Place a cotton wool pad next to the scalp. With a dampened cotton wool pad, wipe the solution evenly across the weft so that it penetrates through the weft and onto the natural hair.

2 Using a hairdryer, heat the weft at the root area for three minutes. Heat activates the removal solution, breaking down the cold-fusion adhesive.

3 Once the adhesive is softened, the weft is ready to peel off. Remove the weft carefully, re-applying removal solution where necessary.

STEP-BY-STEP: COLD-FUSION ADHESIVE TAPE STRIP REMOVAL

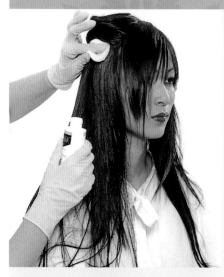

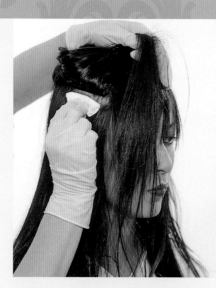

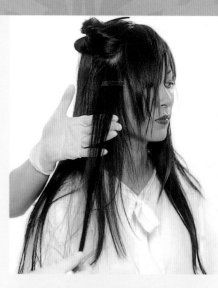

1 Pour a small amount of removal solution onto a cotton wool pad. Wipe the top side of the tape near the root area then lift the tape weft and wipe the underside.

2 Allow the removal solution to penetrate the treated area for 30 to 60 seconds.

3 Hold the end of the extension hair contained in the tape and gently pull it away from the scalp. The weft should glide away from the natural hair.

SUMMARY

Now you have finished this chapter you should have a clearer picture of all the essential aspects associated with assisting with hair extension services. In particular, you should now have a good understanding and be able to:

✓ prepare the client and their hair correctly before the removal service

✓ describe a variety of different hair extension systems and the products and tools associated with each system

✓ explain the maintenance requirements for a variety of different extension systems

✓ carry out the removal of hair extensions for a range of different hot and cold bonding techniques.

In addition, you now understand how these processes will enable you to work more efficiently and effectively in hair extension services.

REVISION QUESTIONS

Q1. Copy and complete this sentence: A removal solution is a chemical formulated to _____ the adhesive connecting the hair extension to the hair.

Fill in the blank

Q2. Cold-fusion hair extensions are a system of connecting hair extensions by using heated resin.

True or False

Q3. What are the four main techniques for bonding extensions to hair? (Choose four answers.)

grafting	☐	a
hot-bonded	☐	b
cold-fusion	☐	c
sewing	☐	d
plaiting	☐	e
twisting	☐	f

Q4. Cold-fusion systems use adhesives, solutions and tapes to hold strands or wefts of extension hair in place on natural hair.

True or False

Q5. A removal tool is used for which type of hair extensions? (Choose one answer.)

cold-fusion systems	○	a
hot-bonded systems	○	b
sewn weft systems	○	c
self-adhesive strands	○	d

10 Assist with Colouring Services

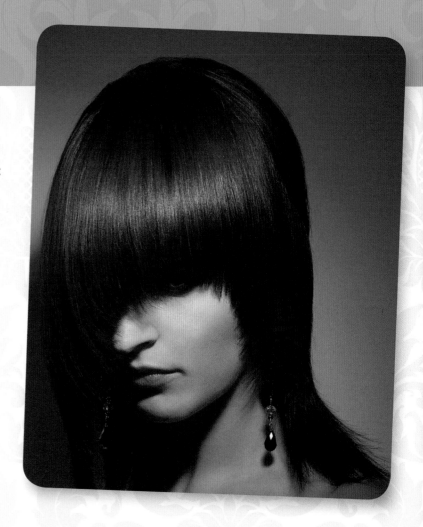

LEARNING OBJECTIVES

When you have finished this chapter you should:

◆ be able to work safely when assisting with colouring services

◆ be able to remove colouring and lightening products

◆ know the products, equipment and their use

◆ know your salon's policies and legal obligations

◆ know how to work safely and hygienically when assisting with colouring services.

KEY TERMS

antioxidant conditioner

dermatitis

emulsify

eumelanin

melanin

permanent colour

pheomelanin

pigment

PPD (para-phenylenediamine)

quasi-permanent colour (tone-on-tone)

semi-permanent colour

skin test

temporary colour

trichosiderin

virgin hair

INFORMATION COVERED IN THIS CHAPTER

PRACTICAL SKILLS

Learn how to work safely and efficiently at all times.

Learn how to work with different colouring products and techniques.

Learn how to remove different colouring processes correctly.

Learn how to apply simple colouring techniques.

UNDERPINNING KNOWLEDGE

Know your salon's ranges of products and services.

Understand the factors that can affect the way that colours need to be removed.

Know the different products associated with the services.

Know the principles of application for different colouring services

Know how to communicate effectively and professionally.

INTRODUCTION

A colouring service can be quick and simple or a complex, in-depth technical process. It covers a variety of different methods for changing a client's hair colour, some of which you might be applying under the supervision of the stylist, and other processes that take a lot longer.

Creating something artistic is not just the stylist's job – you are equally important to the process. The correct removal of colours and particularly the multi-coloured effects of highlighting are critical to achieving a successful result. This chapter helps you understand the differences between colours and lighteners and explains how you can contribute to colouring services.

Natural and synthetic (artificial) hair colour

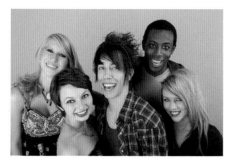

Look at a group of friends – how many colours of hair can you see?

When we look at the natural colour of hair, what we are really seeing are microscopic **pigments** scattered about like grains of sand within the hair's cortex. The natural hair pigments are collectively called **melanin**, and the quantities of these pigments (**eumelanin**, **pheomelanin** and **trichosiderin**) vary between individuals, giving us the natural colour of our hair. Eumelanin produces black or brown pigments and pheomelanin gives yellow and red ones. The naturally occurring colours that you see in hair are a mixture of these two pigments. A third type of pigment called trichosiderin is rare but gives rich 'Celtic red' tones to hair.

The appearance of these natural pigments can be changed or modified temporarily or permanently. Hair colour can be changed by the addition of artificial pigments through the application of colour, or by reduction – the removal of colour, through lightening processes.

Types of synthetic colour

Temporary colour   Temporary colours can produce subtle or bold colour effects. They are available in many forms – setting lotions, mousses, gels, hairsprays, hair mascara, crayons, paints and glitter dust. Temporary colours remain on the cuticle surface of the hair and are ideal for a client try-out colour, as they only last for one shampoo. However, if they are used on badly damaged or very porous hair, the temporary colour may quickly be absorbed into the cortex, producing long-lasting, uneven, patchy results.

HEALTH & SAFETY

It is important to check manufacturer's instructions and your salon policy before undertaking colouring services on anyone under 16 years of age.

- Temporary colours only last for one wash in good conditioned hair.

- They are often difficult to remove from hair that is damaged, porous or lightened.

- You cannot lighten hair with temporary colours.

- You cannot achieve a specific target shade in the same way as you can with longer lasting or permanent colours.

- They may not give you an even coverage on the hair.

- They do not require an allergy alert test 48 hours beforehand.

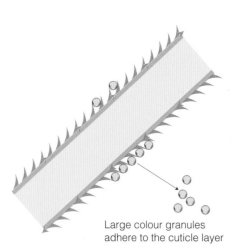

Large colour granules adhere to the cuticle layer

Temporary colours have large colour molecules that sit on the outside of the hair and get trapped in the cuticle layers

Semi-permanent colour   Semi-permanent colours are ideal for clients who want colour but do not want it to last very long. They last for up to six or eight shampoos and do not produce any visible regrowth. The hair loses colour on each shampoo so the effect fades over time. They do not lighten hair; they can only add tones to the existing colour. They contain conditioning agents that add shine and improve style manageability while the colour processes. They can also darken the hair.

Quasi-permanent colour   Quasi-permanent colours are also known as **tone-on tone-colours**. They last longer than semi-permanents but not as long as true permanent colour. They are mixed with a lower strength hydrogen peroxide and also produce regrowth. They will cover some grey hair and are a popular colour choice for people who colour their hair themselves.

Permanent colour

Permanent colours make up the largest variety of shades and tones. They can cover grey (which is in fact white hair) and modify the natural pigments in the hair to produce a range of natural, fashion and fantasy shades. Hydrogen peroxide is mixed with permanent colour to develop the process, and the hair will then retain the colour permanently within the cortex. Hair in poor condition, however, will not hold the colour and colouring could result in patchy areas and colour fading.

Lightener

Lighteners and bleaches contain alkaline chemicals that dissolve the natural pigments in hair. Lightening products are mixed with hydrogen peroxide. They are used in three main forms: high lift colour, powder bleach and oil bleach.

> **TOP TIP**
>
> Never ignore the result of an allergy alert test. If a skin test shows a reaction and you carry on anyway, there may be a more serious reaction that could affect the whole body.

Allergy alert test

STEP-BY-STEP: ALLERGY ALERT TEST

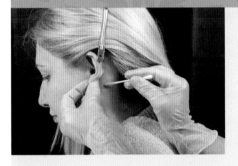 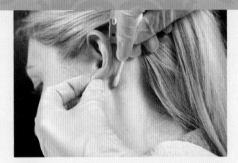 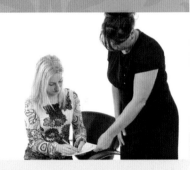

1 Apply a small amount of a dark colour on a cotton bud to a clean area of skin about 5mm square, behind the ear. Always follow the manufacturer's explicit instructions to ensure the salon is covered by their insurance.

2 Do not cover the area; ask your client to report any discomfort or irritation that occurs over the next 48 hours.

3 Record the details on the client's record file (it may be useful for future reference). Get the client to sign to say they have received the Allergy Alert Test and advice regarding any adverse reactions.

HEALTH & SAFETY

Allergy alert tests – Testing for allergies

Permanent and quasi-permanent colours contain a chemical compound called **PPD (para-phenylenediamine)**. This is a known allergen and some people can have a severe allergic reaction to it if it comes into contact with the skin. For this reason, anyone planning a permanent or quasi-permanent colour must have an allergy alert test 48 hours *before* a permanent colouring service.

To carry out an allergy alert test on a client prior to the planned service:

1. Clean an area of skin about 5mm square behind the ear.
2. Select a small amount of a dark colour within the range to be used, on a cotton bud (follow the manufacturer's explicit details).
3. Apply a little of the colour directly to the skin.
4. Do not cover the area and ask your client to report any discomfort or irritation that occurs over the next 48 hours. Arrange to see your client at the end of this time so that you can check for signs of reaction.
5. Record the details on the client's record file (it may be useful for future reference).
6. Make an appointment for the future service.
7. If there is a positive response – a contra-indication such as inflammation, soreness, swelling, irritation or discomfort – do not carry out the intended service.
8. If the result is negative, i.e. no reaction, the service may proceed as planned.

Learning about colouring techniques

ACTIVITY

1. What colouring services are offered at your salon/shop?
2. Does your salon have any particular requirements in the way that colours must be taken off?
3. What materials are used for highlighting services?
4. List the services available in your salon and the materials that are used to create the effects in your portfolio.

Stylists use a variety of classic and contemporary methods to colour a client's hair. Some of these are easy for you to remove at the basin, whereas others are quite complex. A stylist may colour hair using the following techniques:

◆ full head colour

◆ slice or spot colour

◆ regrowth colour

◆ cap highlights

◆ T–section or full head highlights.

ACTIVITY

The table below shows the variety of colouring services that are available for clients, but not every salon or shop does them all. Copy the table and complete the missing information for the colouring services that take place in your shop.

Service	Abbreviation used in the appointment system	What has to be prepared before the service?
Regrowth or retouch colour		
Full head colour		
T–section highlights		
Full head highlights		
Cap highlights		
Spot colour		

TOP TIP

All colouring products are chemicals and must be handled in accordance with the manufacturer's instructions. You must wear the correct PPE (non-latex disposable gloves) when handling chemicals.

Colouring processes in the salon

Full head colour   This is an application of semi, quasi, permanent colour or lightener to all of the hair regardless of length. The colour is applied in a certain order so that the client's hair develops to a final, single colour that is even from the root area to the points of the hair. Care must be taken to **emulsify** the colour so that it releases the colour from the hair, making it easier to shampoo and remove.

Regrowth colour   Regrowth colour, also called a retouch, refers to the application of permanent colour or lightener to the hair that has regrown since the last colour application. It is a line or band of natural hair between the scalp and the artificial/synthetic hair colour. Regrowth colours are fairly simple to remove. They are a single colour applied to only part of the head. Like full head colours, they should be emulsified so that the colour removal provides a better result.

T–section and full head highlights   T–section highlights are a popular way of placing highlights along the parting area and down around the sides of the front hairline. They are usually an in-between option for a client who has a regrowth of natural hair, with highlights still showing within the lengths.

Full head highlights are also a popular technique for creating a multi-toned effect throughout the client's hair. Each meche or foil is carefully positioned so that only the parts requiring colour are processed. The meches keep the colours from merging into the rest of the hair and creating an unwanted and potentially damaging result.

For both highlighting services, the hairstyle may be created through lightening some areas and colouring others. Because of this multi-toning effect, special care needs to be taken during removal so that the (or each individual) colour is carefully removed and is prevented from discolouring other parts of the hair, which creates an unpleasant muddy result.

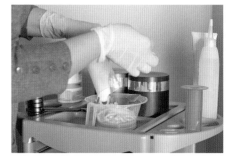
Mixing colours on a trolley

Slice and spot colouring   Slice colouring is very similar to highlights, where sections of hair are taken and coloured to produce more striking, dramatic results. Again, the meches or foils keep the colours from merging into the rest of the hair.

Spot colouring is a technique using temporary semi, quasi, permanent colours or lighteners in specific areas in between regrowth or full head colouring. It is often used for colouring white hair that shows in a parting.

The hair may be lightened and/or coloured. Care needs to be taken removing this type of colour so that each individual colour is carefully removed and is prevented from discolouring other parts of the hair.

Cap highlights   Cap highlights are a way of producing a uniform highlighted result by pulling sections of hair through a rubber cap and applying colour or lightener. The process is a way of producing a single colour effect. This is a simple and popular option for men's colouring. Providing that the cap is not worn and the holes have not split, the removal of cap highlights is fairly simple. After rinsing, make sure that you lift the flange edge back over the cap all round so that the cap comes away easily without too much lugging. It helps to apply conditioner to the hair before removing the cap.

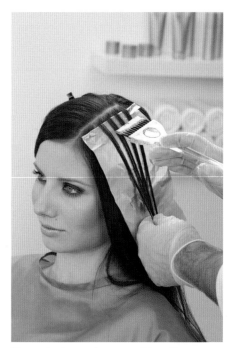
Slice colouring produces a striking effect.

TOP TIP

When you remove the hair colour, make sure that the client is protected and take particular care not to get any water or colouring products on the client's skin or clothes. Any staining is unprofessional and damage to clothes will have to be paid for by the salon!

Remove colour from different services and processes

Work safely while providing services to clients

Preparation is important for any technical process – for colouring it is essential. Consult Chapters 2 and 6 for more information on practices that are common to all services.

HEALTH & SAFETY

Any contact with chemical products is hazardous to health. Avoid developing dermatitis by always wearing disposable gloves.

ACTIVITY

Write your answers to the following questions in your portfolio.

1. What is your salon's policy for protecting clients during colouring services?
2. What PPE is available for clients?
3. What PPE is available for you and when should you wear it?
4. What arrangements does your salon have for the disposal of waste items?
5. How would you know if a client was comfortable or not?

Disposal of waste   Colouring products create a lot of waste in and around the basin area. Unused, leftover colour or lightener should be washed out of colouring bowls as soon as the stylist has finished the service. These products swell up if left for any period of time and therefore need to be thoroughly rinsed away, as they form a sludge that might block the drains. Used foils and meches should be disposed of properly – your salon will have its own procedures for this.

TOP TIP

Never remove all the foils at the same time. Ask the stylist for the correct order in which the colours must be removed.

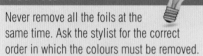

CourseMate video: Removal of capped highlights

Minimizing the risk of hair damage

Different colouring products work in different ways, so removing colours is not as straightforward as you might think. Different colour processes need to be handled differently and this is especially true when two or more colours are to be removed. Lack of care and attention will ruin the result. You must know what to do and understand what is being done before attempting any colour removal. When hair has been coloured and lightened it is in a far more delicate state than normal. You need to be particularly careful when you remove:

◆ highlight caps – apply surface conditioner to the highlights after rinsing and then gently comb through to reduce or eliminate stretching and reduce damage to the client's hair

◆ foils – highlighting foils are folded and cannot be pulled out of the hair without unfolding; you must carefully unfold them separately and rinse the colouring product on each one

◆ meche or colour wraps – some meches (i.e. Easi-meche™) have a sticky edge that bonds on to the hair; these must not be pulled away from the lengths of the hair – they must be individually unwrapped and rinsed before they can be peeled away from the hair.

ACTIVITY

Check your salon's procedure for maintaining stock levels of products and the ways in which the records are completed. Write this information in your portfolio for future reference.

Colouring fault	Action to take
Colour on the client's skin.	Remove with hair colour stain remover at the earliest possible moment.
Colour bleeding out of foils or meche on to other areas.	Tell the stylist immediately so they can take corrective measures.
Colour not taken off properly.	It may continue to develop or will affect any other following services – you must re-shampoo and condition.
Lightener or colour splashed onto the client or in their eyes.	Give the client a dampened cotton wool wad and get help from a senior member of staff immediately.
Lightener or colour splashed onto the colouring gown.	If possible, carefully replace the client's gown with a clean, fresh one; otherwise, sponge the stained area.

Emulsifying the colour

A shampoo will not spread evenly over the colour until it has been mixed with water; it releases the colour from the hair far easier after it has been emulsified. After adjusting the temperature, a small amount of water is sprinkled over the colour then, using the fingertips in a rotary massage technique, the colour is blended together to form an emulsion. The massage is continued as this starts to release the residual colour from the hair, which can then be rinsed away.

For more information on preventing infection, avoiding dermatitis and personal health and hygiene, see Chapter 3 Health and safety.

STEP-BY-STEP: REMOVAL OF LIGHTENING PRODUCT (CAPPED HIGHLIGHTS)

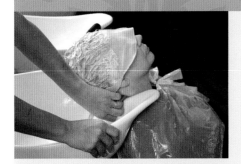

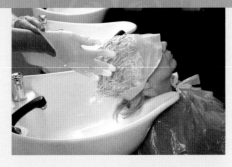

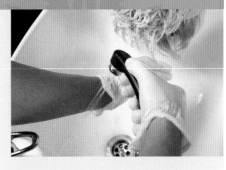

1 Sit the client comfortably at the basin while the highlight cap is still on. Place a freshly laundered towel around the neck and across the shoulders.

2 Put on your disposable gloves and lift the rim of the highlight cap so it isn't caught in the basin.

3 Turn on the water and control the mixture of hot and cold. Test the temperature on the back of the hand to make sure it is neither too cold nor too hot.

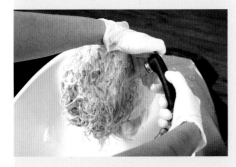

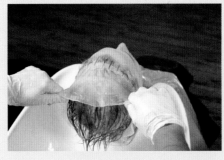

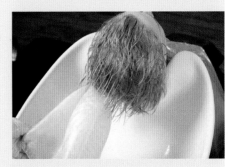

4 Start rinsing the hair while shielding the forehead, down either side, cupping the ears and through to the lengths. Check the flow of water pressure and temperature regularly.

5 Once the product has been rinsed off, apply conditioner to the lightened hair over the cap. This allows the cap to be gently removed without pulling on the hair.

6 Once the cap has been removed, rinse thoroughly and then shampoo and condition the whole head as you would for any other service.

Removing colour

STEP-BY-STEP: REMOVAL OF LIGHTENING PRODUCT (PACKET HIGHLIGHTS)

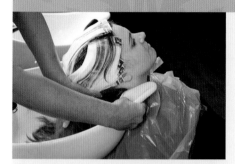

1 Sit the client at the basin, leaving the packets to fall back into the basin. Place a freshly laundered towel around the neck and across the shoulders.

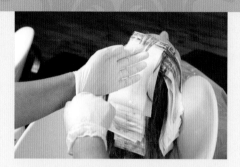

2 Put on your disposable gloves and apron. Turn on the water and control the mixture of hot and cold, testing the temperature on the back of your hand.

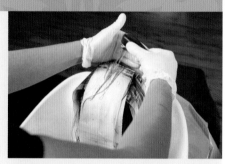

3 Shield the client's face and start rinsing the hair from the forehead, down either side, cupping the ears and through to the lengths. Check the flow of water pressure and temperature regularly.

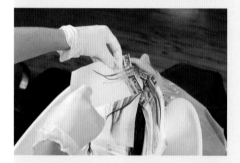

4 Rinse the hair over the packets, gently releasing them from the hair one by one. Remove and dispose of all the packets.

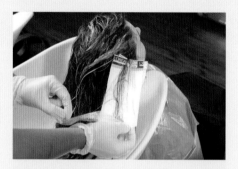

5 You may need to open individual packets and gently release the hair by hand, to prevent the packets from tugging.

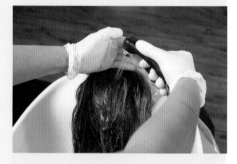

6 Once all the packets have been removed, shampoo and condition the whole head and rinse thoroughly.

TOP TIP

Remember to keep the work area clean and tidy at all times. All waste items should be removed from the sinks and side area. This includes colouring foils, Easi-meche™ colour wraps, etc. Also remove neck wool, plastic caps and plastic capes, and any loose hair caught in the hair traps in the basins.

Removing multiple colours

The removal of highlights, lowlights and slice colouring from the hair is more complex. If two or more colours are introduced to the hair they will be packaged separately in some way. There are special reasons for this:

◆ Different colours need to be kept apart so that they do not merge together, forming an unwanted effect.

◆ Different colours often develop at different rates and therefore some might have been removed earlier than others.

◆ The colouring technique involves specific positioning or placement; this maximizes colour impact by using the shape, texture and style of the hair.

◆ Sometimes the client's hair colour needs correction, perhaps because of a previous poor application or because it has discoloured.

STEP-BY-STEP: REMOVAL OF PERMANENT COLOUR

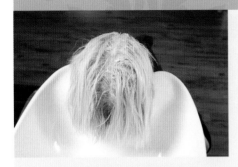

1 Adjust the basin and sit the client back comfortably. Put on your disposable gloves and apron.

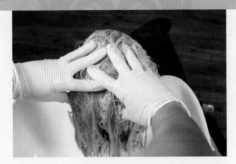

2 Test the temperature of the water on the inside of your wrist and then apply water to the hair. Massage the scalp to lift off the product.

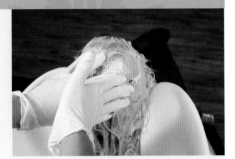

3 Notice how the water mixes with the colour to form an emulsion. Colours come off the scalp easier if they are emulsified first.

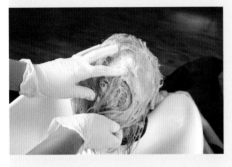

4 Make sure you thoroughly massage the base of the neck and all around the hairline to lift all product out of the hair.

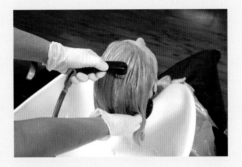

5 Rinse the hair clean, then shampoo twice.

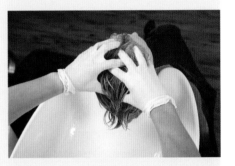

6 Rinse all traces of shampoo lather away from the hair and lightly squeeze out the excess water. Condition the hair with an **antioxidant conditioner**.

You need to know how to recognize different colours within the hair and how to remove them carefully and safely. Generally, for highlights or slice colouring with lighter and darker shades, remove the darkest shade first, then the next darkest and so on, because darker colours may run into lighter hair and ruin the effect. Bleach is sometimes used to lighten hair and, during highlighting, certain areas can develop more readily than others, so some sections will need to be removed earlier than others. The most important thing to remember is if you do not know, ask. There will be a reason for colours to be removed in a specific order.

CourseMate video: Removal of permanent colour

CourseMate video: Removal of packet highlights

Apply conditioners and complete the service

> Salon routines involving the work area are common throughout the Level 1 procedures. Please review this information by turning to Chapter 2 Preparing for work for more information.

> For more information about the indicators of hair in good condition, see Chapter 6 Shampoo and Condition Hair.

TOP TIP

Never attempt to put colour-removing shampoo onto the hair before rinsing with water and emulsifying the product on the hair.

ACTIVITY

Choose the correct answer to each of the following questions.

1. Why should you emulsify the colour before shampooing off?

   A   it saves shampoo

   B   it saves conditioner

   C   it makes it easier to remove

   D   it makes it stay on the hair better

2. When removing highlights, which colours are normally removed first?

   A   the mid-tone colour

   B   the darkest colour

   C   the lightest colour

   D   all at the same time

3. When removing highlights, which colours are normally removed last?

   A   the mid-tone colour

   B   the darkest colour

   C   the lightest colour

   D   all at the same time

4. What effect do you think the addition of bleach will have in a set of highlights?

   A   it makes the hair lighter

   B   it makes the hair darker

   C   it makes the hair blue

   D   it makes the hair white

5. Which product is easier to rinse out of the hair?

   A   semi-permanent colour

   B   permanent colour

   C   bleach

   D   high-lift tint

6. Who decides when a colour is ready for removal?

   A   you

   B   the stylist

   C   the manufacturer

   D   the client

Applying suitable conditioners

Depending on the type of colour used, you should now apply a suitable conditioner to improve the handling of the client's hair and smooth down the cuticle layer.

The oxidation process that takes place during permanent colouring needs to be stopped. This is done using an antioxidant conditioner. These are special conditioners that remove excess oxygen, which is released by the hydrogen peroxide during the colour service. If this residual oxygen is not removed, the free edges of the cuticle may not close down properly and may allow the newly introduced colour pigments to fade prematurely, so the colour will not last.

Leaving the client ready for further services

After completing the shampoo and conditioning processes, you should bring the client into an upright position and show them to a free styling unit. When they are seated, remove the towel and gently detangle the hair with a wide-tooth comb. Finally, squeeze any excess moisture from the hair and tell the stylist that their client is ready. It is courteous to offer the client a drink at this point.

SUMMARY

Now you have finished this chapter you should have a clearer picture of all the essential aspects associated with assisting with colouring and lightening services. In particular, you should now have a good understanding and be able to:

✓ prepare the client and their hair correctly before the colouring or lightening service

✓ describe the differences between natural and artificial hair colour

✓ describe the different types of artificial colour and understand in basic terms how they affect natural hair

✓ recognize the types of colour that require an allergy alert test and know the procedures for conducting this test for clients prior to their appointment

✓ apply certain types of colour in accordance with the stylist's explicit instructions

✓ remove certain types of colour in accordance with the stylist's explicit instructions

✓ work safely at all times during colouring services and processes.

In addition, you now understand how these principles and processes will enable you to work more efficiently and effectively in daily salon routines.

REVISION QUESTIONS

Q1. Copy and complete this sentence: A semi-permanent colour will _____ during shampooing.

Fill in the blank

Q2. Natural hair that has not been coloured is called **virgin hair**.

True or False

Q3. Which of the following are natural pigments found within the hair? (You may choose more than one answer.)

paraphenylenediamine ☐ a

pheomelanin ☐ b

eumelanin ☐ c

alpha keratin ☐ d

beta keratin ☐ e

henna ☐ f

Q4. A lightener will remove natural pigments in hair.

True or False

Q5. Which of the following colours does not produce a regrowth? (Choose one answer.)

semi-permanent ○ a

quasi-permanent ○ b

permanent ○ c

lightener ○ d

11 Assist with Perming Services

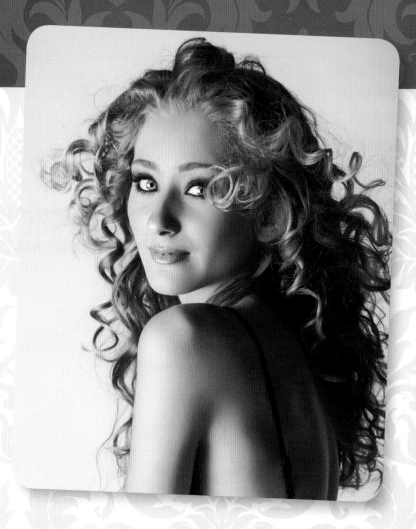

LEARNING OBJECTIVES

When you have finished this chapter you should:

◆ be able to work safely when assisting with perming services

◆ be able to apply perming products

◆ be able to neutralize hair after perming services

◆ know the products, equipment and their use

◆ know your salon's policies and legal obligations

◆ know how to work safely and hygienically when assisting with perming services.

KEY TERMS

ammonium thioglycolate

antioxidant conditioner

disulphide bonds

fish-hooks

neutralizer

pH level

post damping

INFORMATION COVERED IN THIS CHAPTER

PRACTICAL SKILLS

Learn how to work safely and efficiently at all times.

Learn how to work with different perming products and processes.

Learn how to prepare for perming and neutralizing services.

Learn how to neutralize hair correctly.

UNDERPINNING KNOWLEDGE

Know your salon's range of products and services.

Understand the factors that can affect the results of a perm during neutralizing.

Know the different products associated with the services.

Know how to apply solutions for different perming and neutralizing treatments.

Know how to communicate effectively and professionally.

INTRODUCTION

Perming is a complex process and a satisfactory result can only be achieved if all sequences in the process are carried out correctly. The first part depends on the care and attention of the stylist when they:

◆ choose the correct size curlers for the result required

◆ place the curlers in the correct way to achieve the lift and degree of movement required

◆ select the correct lotion matched to the needs of the hair

◆ develop the perm to the point where the optimum result is achieved.

However, these techniques can be ruined if the second part of the process is not carried out properly, and this is where your careful assistance is crucial.

Work safely while providing services to clients

Basic science – how do perms work?

The chemical reactions that take place within the hair during perming involve some complex chemistry that is covered in NVQ Levels 2 and 3. However, a simpler way of explaining the changes that take place within the hair during perming and neutralizing is to use an illustration:

If you imagine that a ladder represents a single hair, the strength of the ladder is in the two long uprights. However, when you climb the ladder it flexes. Therefore, although it is strong and rigid, it is also capable of movement. The strength and shape of the ladder is derived from the rungs. Each rung is evenly spaced, holding the main structure of long uprights apart. These rungs are like the **disulphide bonds** in the hair shaft; they give natural hair its strength.

During perming, a solution of **ammonium thioglycolate** is added to the hair after the curlers have been wound in. The solution breaks the disulphide bonds chemically, just as if you had taken a saw and cut through all the rungs. Therefore, if you imagine that the ladder is now bent, the rungs now do not line up in the same places; the cut rungs have changed positions.

The next part of the perming process – neutralizing – re-fixes the bonds by adding a solution enriched with oxygen. Just like the bent ladder, the rungs are now glued together in a new, reformed shape and, just like perming, if the gluing is done well the ladder remains in a permanently bent shape. If it is done poorly, the ladder springs back to a straighter shape.

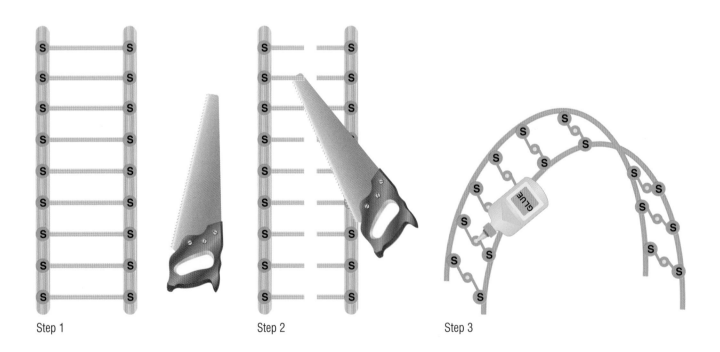

Step 1   Step 2   Step 3

The illustrations on page 186 help to explain it in another way:

1. The ladder represents the hair and disulphide bonds as rungs holding the ladder together.

2. When perm lotion is applied, the rungs/disulphide bonds are broken.

3. During perming, the hair is bent around a curler. The disulphide bonds are then re-formed in the neutralizing process, into their new locations; permanently waving the hair.

Correctly protect and position the client and yourself

Gowning the client Because perm solutions are generally applied to hair by **post damping** (a method of pre-winding a perm and then applying the perm lotion after), the solutions tend to be very watery. This could be a hazard to the client, particularly if it is spilt on them or too much is applied and it runs down around their face and neck.

TOP TIP

Dermatitis is an occupational hazard for hairdressers. you can reduce the risk by wearing vinyl or nitrile gloves when using chemicals, which provide you with a guaranteed barrier against the action of harsh chemicals on the skin.

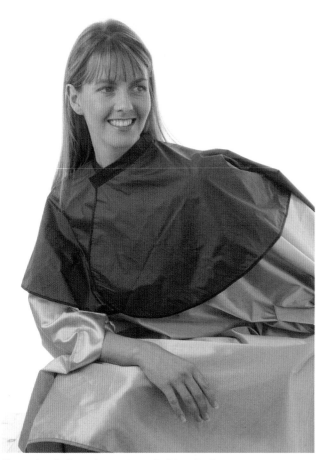

Use a chemical-proof gown topped with a plastic cape

BEST PRACTICE

Barrier cream can be applied around the client's hairline before the perm is applied. It will help to prevent harm from chemicals during processing.

Perm solutions are alkaline with a pH 8.5 – 9, and if lotion makes contact with the skin and is not removed it could cause irritation, swelling and even chemical burns. If it gets on the client's clothes it will probably discolour the fabric. Therefore, make sure that the client is well protected. Put on a chemical-proof gown and secure a clean, fresh towel into place around their shoulders. Fix a plastic cape on top, ensuring that it is comfortable around the neck. Mop up any perm lotion spills with cotton wool/neck wool.

Work safely while providing services to clients (Continued...)

Protecting yourself

Your salon will provide all the personal protective equipment (PPE) that you may need in routine daily practices. Perming involves the handling and application of chemicals, so you must protect yourself from their potentially hazardous effects. Always read the manufacturer's instructions and follow the methods of practice that they specify. You are expected to wear and use the PPE provided for you. In the case of perming, these include disposable vinyl or nitrile gloves and a water/splash-proof apron.

TOP TIP

Your salon will have its own way of neutralizing that will be suited to the products it uses. Find out what it is and how you are expected to do it.

Your posture   Neutralizing takes a lot longer than shampooing so your standing position is particularly important. Review the sections on back and side wash positions in Chapter 6, Shampoo and condition hair, so that you know and can avoid the risk of injury or a longer term back condition.

ACTIVITY

The Control of Substances Hazardous to Health (COSHH) Regulations 2003 explain the potential risks that hairdressing chemicals can have. Read the manufacturer's instructions for safe handling, storage and disposal in your salon. Perming products should be stored in an upright position and in a cool, dry place away from strong sunlight. Find out what the arrangements are in your salon and write these down in your portfolio for future reference.

For more information on preventing infection, avoiding dermatitis and personal health and hygiene, see Chapter 3 Health and safety.

ACTIVITY

Answer these 'true or false' questions:

◆ Neutralizer is used in a perm service to fix wave into hair – true or false?

◆ You should always follow manufacturer's instructions when mixing chemicals – true or false?

◆ Neutralizer is applied before rinsing – true or false?

◆ Wearing disposable gloves helps to avoid developing dermatitis – true or false?

Keep work areas clean and safe to use at all times

Remove and dispose of waste items as soon as possible. Do not leave cotton, neck wool, plastic caps, etc. around the basins; put them into a covered bin. Wash, dry and replace perm curlers back into the trays as soon as possible. Perming chemicals should be applied in a well-ventilated area. If there is any waste (some perming solutions cannot be saved for use another time), flush it down the basin with plenty of cold water.

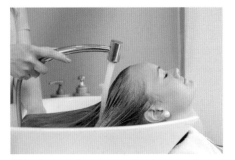

All businesses have metered water – running water down the drain costs money!

Minimize waste   Get into the habit of eliminating waste. All the resources that you use cost money and the only way that you can be more effective is to maximize your time and efforts while minimizing the cost of carrying out your work.

Water is a costly but essential part of hairdressing, and all business premises have metered water. Therefore, in principle, every shampoo and conditioning rinse can be a calculated cost. Rinsing for longer than necessary or leaving taps running between shampoos incurs unnecessary costs, especially if the water is hot.

Reporting low stocks of neutralizing product

You are responsible for the neutralizing process and you will be the first to notice when neutralizers are running low or containers have been left with their tops off. The success of the perm is directly related to the chemical reaction of the neutralizer, so if too little or a defective product is used, then the perm will not work. Look at the condition and quantities of the products in stock and if the salon or shop is running low, tell someone who is responsible for stock reordering.

Be efficient and effective with your time

- Always make good use of your time. There are always things to do in and around the salon or shop.

- Clean work areas so that they are ready to receive clients.

- Prepare materials, look out for stock shortages and report them.

- Prepare the equipment – cleaning and washing the brushes, combs and curlers.

- Prepare client records and get things ready for when they arrive.

- Prepare the trolleys, get the right curlers ready, make sure that the rubbers have not perished and the end papers are at hand.

Choosing a neutralizer

Manufacturers match their perms to their neutralizers. They are designed to work together and chemically balance each other out during the process. Always use the correct lotions – many perms are now individually packed and you will find a perm lotion and its matched neutralizer in the box.

TOP TIP

Perming products are chemically matched to the quantity and strengths of the neutralizing solutions. If there is insufficient product the perm will fail. If the top of the neutralizer has been left off, the solution will be too weak to work properly.

ACTIVITY

Answer the following questions in your portfolio:

1 Why is neutralizer an essential part to the perming process?

2 Why is timing a critical factor in the neutralizing process?

TOP TIP

When you have a spare moment in the salon, separate the perm curlers into their different colour sizes. Check the condition of the perm rubbers and replace those that have perished or have become over-elastic. When you have washed and dried them, separate them into bundles of nine with a tenth curler around them, binding them together. You have now sorted the trolley trays into easily managed sizes and numbers!

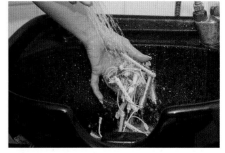

Rinsing perming curlers after the neutralizing process

Neutralizing hair

Neutralizing (rebalancing the hair)

Neutralizing is the process of fixing the curl or movement into the hair and returning it to a balanced chemical state. An industry term, 'neutralizing' is a little misleading. In chemistry, a 'neutral' chemical condition is neither acidic nor alkaline (pH 7.0). However, in hairdressing, the neutralizing treatment returns the previously processed hair to the natural state of pH 5.5. (For more information about pH values see Chapter 6 page 113.)

Preparing the neutralizer properly

Neutralizing always takes place at the basin, so any plastic caps, capes or cotton wool must be carefully removed and any damp towels must be replaced. To prepare, first gather the materials you need and then make sure there is a backwash basin free.

Rinsing perm lotion from hair

Rinsing thoroughly with warm water removes the perming chemicals from the hair and stops any further processing. When you rinse you must take special care not to dislodge any of the curlers or rods.

First rinsing

1. As soon as the perm is complete, move the client immediately to the backwash basin. Make sure they are comfortable.

2. Carefully remove the cap. The hair is in a soft and weak stage at this point, so do not put unnecessary tension on it. Leave the curlers in place.

3. Run the water. You need an even supply of warm water. The water must be neither hot nor cold, as this will be uncomfortable for the client. Hot water will also irritate the scalp and could burn. Check the pressure and temperature against the back of your hand. Remember that your client's head may be sensitive after the perming process.

4. Rinse the hair thoroughly with warm water. This may take about five minutes, or longer if the hair is long. It is this rinsing that stops the perm process – until you rinse away the lotion, the hair will still be processing. Direct the water away from the client's eyes and face.

5. Make sure you rinse all the client's hair, including the nape curlers. If a curler slips out, gently wind the hair back onto it immediately. Be methodical to ensure no curlers are missed. Use your hand to direct the water and prevent it running down in front of the client's ears.

Applying the neutralizer correctly

After rinsing, blot the saturated hair with a dry towel until it is slightly damp. Prepare and apply the correct neutralizer (following the manufacturer's instructions) and leave on for the appropriate length of time.

BEST PRACTICE

Rebalancing the **pH level** of the hair is essential for maintaining hair in good condition. If the hair is not rebalanced it will be dry and porous, and the perm will be very difficult to manage afterwards.

TOP TIP

Check that the client is comfortable and that towels support the client's neck and form a barrier, preventing water from running down the back of their neck. Backwash basins are preferable because it is easier to keep the chemicals away from the client's eyes.

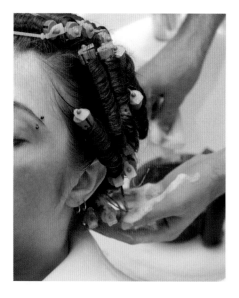

STEP-BY-STEP: APPLYING NEUTRALIZER

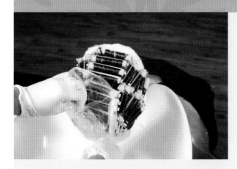

1 Take the client to the basin, making sure they sit in a comfortable position with their head tilted back. Remove the cap and cotton wool.

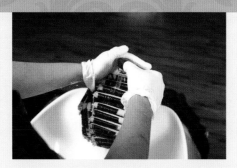

2 Rinse the curlers with warm water, following the manufacturer's instructions. Make sure that you rinse each curler thoroughly.

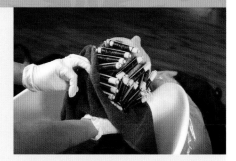

3 Blot the hair thoroughly, using a towel. Then, using the correct neutralizer, follow the manufacturer's instructions for applying to each curler.

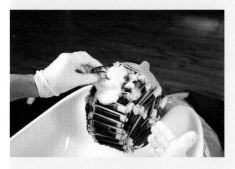

4 Make sure that the neutralizer comes into contact with all the curlers.

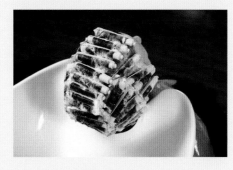

5 When all the hair has been covered, time the process according to the manufacturer's instructions. The usual time is five to ten minutes.

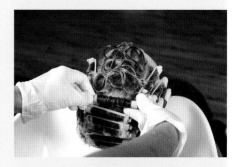

6 After the specified time, carefully remove the curlers. Do not pull or stretch the hair as it may affect the curl formation.

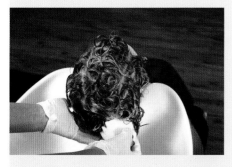

7 Apply the remaining lotion to all the hair. Do not stretch the hair or allow excess lotion to drip down across the client's face. Use cotton wool around the hairline if necessary.

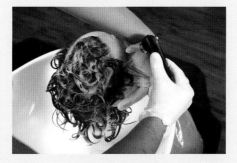

8 Run the water again, checking temperature and pressure. Rinse the hair thoroughly to remove all the neutralizer.

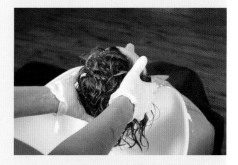

9 To complete the treatment apply an after-perm **antioxidant** conditioner following the manufacturer's instructions.

Applying a suitable conditioner

Perm aids or conditioner and balanced conditioners (antioxidants) help neutralize the effect of the chemical process by helping to restore the pH balance of the hair to pH 5.5. They also smooth down the hair cuticle, improving the hair's look, feel, comb-ability and handling. At the end of the neutralizing process you will have returned the hair to a normal, stable state.

CourseMate video: Neutralizing

After the perm

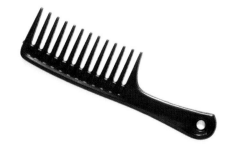

Use a wide-tooth comb to detangle the hair after perming. Start combing the ends of the hair and work up.

Bring the client into an upright position and show them to a free styling unit. When they are seated, remove the towel and gently detangle the hair with a wide-tooth comb. Finally, squeeze any excess moisture from the hair and tell the stylist that their client is ready.

Perming and neutralizing faults

The following table highlights typical problems that can occur during perming and neutralizing. Many of the faults are created in the perming part of the process and have been left in to show how many things can go wrong. However, the possible causes that are created by poor or incorrect neutralizing and not following the manufacturer's instructions are indicated with a star (*). Always tell the stylist if you see or think you have an unexpected result.

Fault	Possible cause
Scalp is tender, sore or broken	Curlers were too tight Wound curlers rested on the skin Lotion was spilt on the scalp * There was cotton wool padding soaked with chemicals between the curlers Hair was pulled tightly Perm was over-processed
Hair is broken	Hair was wound too tightly Curlers were secured too tightly * Incorrect chemicals were used Hair was over-processed Chemicals in the hair reacted with the lotion
Hair is straight	* Wrong neutralizing lotion was used for the type of hair Hair was under-processed Curlers were too large for the hair length * Neutralizing was not done properly * Rinsing was inadequate Conditioners used before perming were still on the hair Hair was coated and resistant to the lotion
Hair is frizzy	Lotion was too strong for hair of this texture Winding was too tight Curlers were too small Hair was over-processed * Neutralizing was not done properly There are fish-hooks
Perm is weak and drops	* Lotion was applied unevenly * Neutralizer was too dilute * Neutralizing was poorly done * Hair was stretched while soft Curlers or sections were too large
Some hair sections are straight	Curler angle was wrong Curlers were placed incorrectly Curlers were too large Sectioning or winding was done carelessly * Neutralizer was not applied correctly

SUMMARY

Now you have finished this chapter you should have a clearer picture of all the essential aspects associated with assisting with perming and neutralizing processes. In particular, you should now have a good understanding and be able to:

✓ prepare the client before perming and neutralizing services

✓ work safely when assisting with perming and neutralizing services

✓ apply perming and neutralizing products

✓ prepare a range of products and equipment for use within the service

✓ work safely and hygienically when assisting with perming services.

In addition, you now understand how these processes enable you to work more efficiently and effectively in perming and neutralizing services.

REVISION QUESTIONS

Q1. Copy and complete this sentence: neutralizer is a chemical that is used to _____ the curl into previously permed hair.

Fill in the blank

Q2. The post-damping method requires the perm to be wound first.

True or False

Q3. Which of the following pH values would indicate acidic properties? (You may choose more than one answer.)

pH 4	☐	a
pH 5	☐	b
pH 6	☐	c
pH7	☐	d
pH8	☐	e
pH9	☐	f

Q4. The COSHH regulations cover the legal requirements for handling chemical products.

True or False

Q5. Which of the following PPE is made available for your benefit? (Choose one answer.)

Gown	○	a
Towel	○	b
Vinyl gloves	○	c
Plastic cape	○	d

12 Assist with Shaving Services

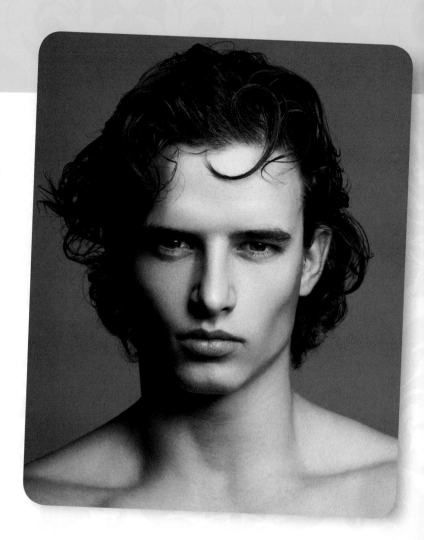

LEARNING OBJECTIVES

When you have finished this chapter you should:

◆ be able to work safely when assisting with shaving services

◆ be able to prepare shaving products, tools and equipment

◆ be able to apply lather in preparation for shaving

◆ know the products, equipment and their uses

◆ know your shop's policies and legal obligations

◆ know how to work safely and hygienically when assisting with shaving services.

KEY TERMS

alum block

badger brush

body odour

brush stand

cut-throat razor

exfoliation

halitosis

moisturizing balms

razor burn

sharps

sharps box

INFORMATION COVERED IN THIS CHAPTER

PRACTICAL SKILLS

Learn how to work safely and hygienically at all times.

Learn how to use and prepare different shaving products, tools and equipment.

Learn how to apply shaving products correctly.

UNDERPINNING KNOWLEDGE

Know your shop's ranges of products and services.

Know how skin reacts to different shaving preparations and lotions.

Know how to work safely and hygienically for shaving services.

Know how to prepare and apply shaving products.

Know how to communicate effectively and professionally.

INTRODUCTION

The purpose of shaving is to remove unwanted hair. Most men consider this daily routine a chore and something that should be carried out as quickly as possible, to free up time for their busy lives. However, it need not be regarded as such, because a good barber can make shaving a relaxing and luxuriant service – one that you will be helping to offer your clients.

Work safely while providing services to clients

You will be using a range of shaving equipment and products. These materials need to be handled safely and made hygienically clean so that they are ready for use. This includes the sterilization of brushes, bowls, etc.

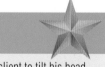

For more information on hygiene and cleaning, see Chapter 3 Health and Safety and Chapter 2 Preparing for Work.

Correctly protect clients and yourself

Gowning the client   Always use fresh, clean, laundered equipment:

◆ Fasten a gown at the back or secure the cutting square with a clip to ensure that the covering is close fitting around the neck and protects the client from any spillages.

◆ Place a towel around the front of the client so that the free edges are fastened at the back.

◆ Tuck a strip of neck wool (or neck tissue) into the top edge of the towel to stop lather and hair fragments from falling inside the client's clothes.

Correctly position clients and yourself

Client posture   The client sits with their head tilted back so you need to work at an angle that enables you to work safely and carefully. If you need to recline the chair, you could do it before the client is seated.

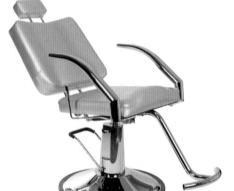

A barber's chair is designed so the client can tilt his head back for shaving

The client's posture should:

◆ allow them to sit comfortably with their back, neck and head fully supported

◆ prevent them from twisting or 'hunching up'

◆ give you the access and freedom to work on and around the client properly and safely.

If you need to make any adjustments to working height or angle, do it before the service is started.

Your working posture   Barbering involves a lot of standing so you will need to be comfortable in your work. You should always adopt a comfortable but safe work position, but sometimes comfortable and safe are not necessarily the same thing. A naturally comfortable position for work should allow you to:

◆ stand close enough to the barber's chair without being supported by it

◆ position your shoulders and torso directly above your hips and feet, with your weight evenly distributed

◆ work without having to twist or bend forwards over the chair.

BEST PRACTICE

Shaving requires the client to tilt his head back so that you can work at an angle that enables you to work safely and carefully. The barber's chair is specifically designed for this, with both its in-built headrest and reclining ability. This ensures the client's comfort and safety.

Shaving position   The client's shaving position and height from the floor have a direct effect on your working position. You must be able to work in a position where everything you need is at hand, i.e. hot towels, lathering products and equipment.

Keeping work areas clean and safe to use at all times

Make good use of your time. Do not leave things to the last minute as this could affect the amount of time available for the barber to do his job. Prepare the tools and equipment so that they are cleaned and sterilized.

Cleanliness is essential – the work area should be clean and free from clutter and waste items; any used materials should be disposed of and not left out on the side. Anything less would be:

- ◆ unprofessional and show that you are disorganized

- ◆ a hazard and present a health risk to others.

You need to be thinking about all of the things that you need *before* you need them.

> **TOP TIP**
>
> Make sure you have your equipment to-hand; this shows that you are organized and it looks more professional too.

ACTIVITY

Answer the following questions in your portfolio:

What is your shop's policy with respect to each of the following practices?

A   The safe disposal of sharp items

B   The cleaning and maintenance of shaving materials

C   Working safely within the shop

D   Preparing the client prior to shaving

> **TOP TIP**
>
> Bad breath is offensive to clients. Bad breath (**halitosis**) is the result of leaving particles to decay within the spaces between the teeth. Brush your teeth after every meal. Bad breath can also result from digestive troubles, stomach upsets, smoking and strong foods such as onion, garlic and some cheeses. Do not smoke when you are on duty.

Maintaining personal hygiene standards

Personal hygiene is vitally important for anyone working in personal services. Your personal hygiene, or lack of it, will be immediately noticeable to everyone you come into contact with. You may have overslept, but if you have not showered it will be very uncomfortable for you, your colleagues and the clients.

Body odour (BO) is unpleasant in any situation and other strong odours are offensive too. The smells of smoking or general bad breath are very off-putting to the client, particularly if they are a non-smoker. Do not smoke at all when you are on duty, not even outside or during comfort breaks.

For more information on personal hygiene see Chapter 3 Health and Safety.

Work safely while providing services to clients (Continued...)

Tool preparation and maintenance

The tools that you use must always be sterilized and ready for use. The materials need to be kept close at hand but well out of the way of clients and children. Any used disposable blades should be disposed of properly in the **sharps box**.

Brushes   The best quality shaving brushes are made of pure badger bristle. The hair for the finest quality brush is taken from the neck of the animal and the natural texture and shape of the individual hairs provide a bristle that is coarse and stiff at the root end while tapering slowly towards a soft, fine tip. Natural badger hair produces a brush that is both durable yet very flexible. There are three quality standards for **badger brushes**:

◆ Pure is a basic brush with short- to medium-length dark hair.

◆ Best has medium- to long-length hairs and a creamy tip; it is slightly softer.

◆ Super is a long-length bristle brush with a creamy tip and has better water retention properties than pure or best quality.

Other brushes are made of synthetic (artificial) materials such as nylon or acrylic.

ACTIVITY

Copy the table below and fill in the missing information.

Sterilizing method	What tools and equipment is it used for?	How does it work?
Barbicide™		
UV cabinet		
Autoclave		

Bowls and mugs   Traditionally, shaving bowls were made of polished chrome metal with a lid, or made of wood. Modern versions are made of alloys or plastics that are lighter to hold and easier to clean and sterilize.

Ceramic mugs are a popular alternative to bowls. Although they do not have the heat retention properties of metal bowls, they do have the benefit of having a handle and are therefore easier and possibly safer to hold when applying lather.

Sponges   Sponges are used for sponge shaving. It is unlikely that you will be involved with assisting during the shave but you will need to know how to prepare and clean them for the barber. Sponges are soaked in hot water and drawn over the face to open the beard follicles just before the razor's blade sweeps over it. This method of shaving is *only* suitable for coarser, heavier growth.

Brush stands   Shaving **brush stands** provide the ideal way of air-drying lathering brushes. Wet brushes are placed on the stand so that the bristles point downwards. This allows the bristles to dry in a naturally straight position and stops the bristles from bending, developing mildew and rotting, therefore prolonging the life of the brush.

Cleaning the equipment

Equipment	Method of cleaning/sterilization
Towels	Large stocks of towels should be machine washed, dried and folded ready for use.
Shaving brush	Wash in hot soapy water, flick dry and place on a brush stand to dry. Before they are used, they can be placed in the UV cabinet for ten minutes.
Shaving bowls	Wash in hot soapy water and dry, then immerse in Barbicide™ or a bath of Cidex™ for 30 minutes. Alternatively, metal items can be sterilized in a UV cabinet or autoclave for 20 minutes.
Shaving mugs	Wash in hot soapy water and dry, then immerse in Barbicide™ or a bath of Cidex™ for 30 minutes. Alternatively, sterilize in a UV cabinet or autoclave for 20 minutes.
Brush stands and shaving brush holders	Wash in hot soapy water and then dry. Metal stands can be placed in an autoclave for 20 minutes; plastic brush holders can be placed in a UV cabinet for 25 minutes.
Sponges	Wash in hot soapy water and immerse in Barbicide™ for 30 minutes.

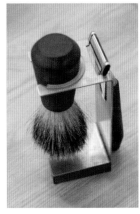

Never stand the brush on its end on the brush stand – the bristles will become misshapen and rot. Always point the bristles downwards

> **TOP TIP**
>
> Always follow the manufacturer's instructions when using or preparing shaving products.

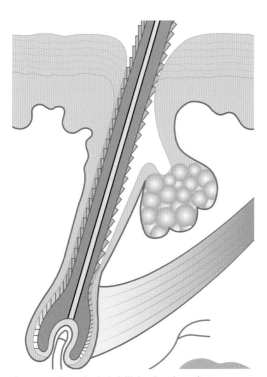

Cross-section of a hair follicle: drawing a hot sponge over the beard will open the follicles and enable a smoother shave

Work safely while providing services to clients (Continued...)

Avoiding cross-infestation and cross-infection

Ultraviolet radiation   Ultraviolet (UV) radiation provides an alternative sterilizing option. The items for sterilization are placed in wall- or worktop-mounted cabinets fitted with UV-emitting light bulbs and exposed to the radiation for at least 15 minutes.

See Chapter 3 Health and safety for more information on preventing infection.

Chemical sterilization   Chemical sterilizers such as Barbicide™ or Cidex™ should be handled only with suitable personal protective equipment (PPE), as many of the solutions used are hazardous to health and should not come into contact with the skin. The most effective form of sterilization is achieved by the total immersion of the contaminated implements into a jar or bath of these fluids.

Autoclave   The autoclave provides a very efficient way of sterilizing using heat. It is particularly good for metal tools – the high temperatures are not suitable for plastic items such as brushes and combs. Items placed in the autoclave take around 20 minutes to sterilize. Check with manufacturers' instructions for variations.

TOP TIP

If your scissors or combs are sterilized in a UV cabinet, remember to turn them over to make sure both sides have been done.

ACTIVITY

Copy the table below into your portfolio and fill in the missing information.

Tools and equipment	How are they cleaned and maintained?
towels	
shaving bowls	
shaving brushes	
brush stands	
sponges	

Dealing with waste and shortages

TOP TIP

Lathering brushes, sponges and bowls must be sterilized after each client.

Safe disposal of waste   There will always be some waste materials at the end of a shave. Sharps must be disposed of in a sharps box. Unused lather should be washed down the sink. It cannot be used again on another client because this may cause cross-infection. Towels need to be laundered and should be removed from the work area or placed into a covered towel bin prior to washing.

TOP TIP

Used razor blades and similar items should be placed into a safe container (sharps box), which must be clearly labelled and the top always re-tightened after disposal. When the container is full it can be disposed of safely. This type of salon waste should be kept away from general salon waste, as there will be special disposal arrangements, possibly provided by your local authority.

Look out for low stocks of materials

Towels   A busy barber's shop will go through a lot of towels during the day. When towel bins are full or when clean stocks are starting to run low, make sure that more towels are put in the washing machine on the appropriate wash cycle. After washing, the towels must be dried and stored ready for use.

Neck strips   Neck strips are tucked in around the collar of gowns or cutting squares to stop bristle fragments falling into the client's clothes. Keep an eye on the neck strip dispenser and replace the roll when it is running low.

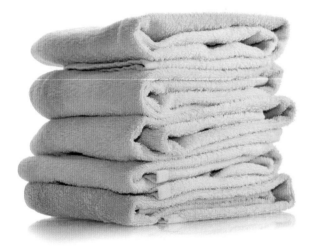

TOP TIP

Barbers use a wide range of products that can be used in the shaving process. Keep an eye on the levels of stock and if you think that items are running low and you cannot find them in stock, tell the person responsible for products so that new stock can be re-ordered.

Learning about shaving products

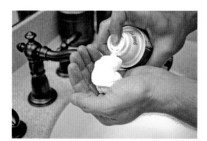

Use shaving foam sparingly - the size of a small orange is normally enough

Shaving oil

Shaving oils contain natural plant oils that moisturize the face while providing the perfect base for a close, comfortable shave. They are particularly suited to those with sensitive skins.

Application   Put 3–4 drops in the palm of your hand and then gently slap both palms together for 1–2 seconds before massaging the oil into the face. Let the oil work its way into the skin for at least one minute before applying the lather. Use this minute to wash the oil from your hands.

Shaving cream

Shaving creams moisturize the skin while providing good lubrication for the shave. Moisturizing shaving creams can be used for all skin types, but normal to drier skins will benefit most from the creams.

Application   The cream is applied prior to the shave. Apply the cream thinly with fingertips to the area to be shaved or lather up with a damp shaving brush and apply to the beard.

Shaving soap

Shaving soap provides the basic lubrication for a good close shave. Moisturizing shaving soaps will create a rich, lubricating lather that softens and moisturizes the skin.

Application   The soap is applied prior to the shave. Apply the cream thinly with fingertips to the area to be shaved or lather up with a damp shaving brush and apply to the beard.

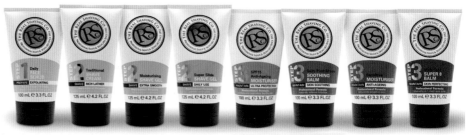

A variety of shaving products to suit different skin types and treatment purposes

Alum block

An **alum block** is a crystal-like stone that is moistened with cold water and gently rubbed over the shaved area to act as an antiseptic for **razor burn**. It can also help to stop bleeding of small nicks and cuts. The alum block also has antiseptic properties that not only cool and refresh the skin after shaving, but also act as a balm.

Application   Simply wet the block, rub gently onto the shaved area and then leave to dry on the face.

Aftershave balm

Shaving balms provide a moisturizing effect that soothes and calms the skin after shaving. **Moisturizing balms** are more suited for dry or sensitive skin types.

Application   Use a dab of the balm and massage gently onto the skin to assist absorption.

Aftershave lotion

Moisturizing lotions replace lost oils and protect, cool and condition the skin after shaving. They are suitable for normal to dry skin types.

Application   Use a dab of the lotion and massage gently or pat onto the skin to assist absorption.

ACTIVITY

Study this table and fill in the missing information.

Product	When is it applied?	How is it applied?
Shaving oil		
Shaving cream		
Shaving soap		
Alum block		
Aftershave balm		
Aftershave lotion		

Preparing the client for shaving

First of all, if the client's bristles are longer than 3mm (the length of a number 1 blade) then they will need to be pre-trimmed with clippers without any attachments fitted. The client's skin is then prepared by cleansing and exfoliation, applying hot towels and then applying the lather.

> **TOP TIP**
>
> An exfoliating face wash will deep clean and prepare the skin for shaving services.

Cleansing and exfoliating the skin

The client's skin can be cleansed by washing with a mild soap or with a granular exfoliating face wash and water. **Exfoliation** is a process that will help remove the layer of dead cells that cover the face and lift the hairs into an upright position.

Applying hot and cold towels

Prepare the skin and beard by applying hot towels to the face to ensure that the lather is applied to a warm face. Hot towels can be prepared by pre-heating in a microwave, a warming cabinet or soaking them in a basin of hot water. After wringing out the excess water they are placed around the facial area, but not covering the nose to:

> **TOP TIP**
>
> Pre-soak towels in a basin of hot water then wring out the excess water and place around the face (do not cover the nose). Hot towels open up the follicles and prepare the skin for massage. Ensure that the towels are not dripping wet and they are not too hot.

- soften the bristly hair
- cleanse the face
- open up the follicles
- prepare the skin for lathering.

Always make sure that the towels are not dripping wet. Check the temperature before applying the towels so that they are hot enough to prepare the skin but not too hot that they burn the client's skin.

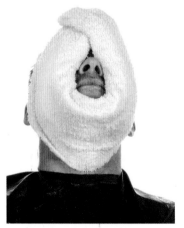

Leave the client's nose free to breathe when covering his face with a hot towel

TOP TIP

Hot towels should not be used on a client with sensitive skin because this will irritate the skin further and prevent you from carrying out the service. Cool towels are used to soothe the face after shaving and to close the pores to finish the service. Cool towels should not be used on a client who is going to have a facial massage because this will close the pores prematurely and prevent the client from gaining the full benefit of the massage service.

Applying lathering products

Traditionally lather was made up from soap and applied with a brush. Now there is a range of lathering products that can be applied by brush.

Lather needs to be applied quickly in a circulatory movement. Take particular care not to go beyond the extent of the beard, as the barber will not be able to see the beard line beneath the lather. Do not cover the mouth, nose or go anywhere near the client's eyes.

Preparing to lather

1. Positioning: Adjusting the chair – recline the barber's chair and adjust the working height (and headrest) so that when you move around the chair you can reach over the client's face without leaning or resting on them.

2. Hygiene: Make sure that your hands are scrupulously clean. Place a clean tissue over the headrest to prevent the spread of infection from one head to another.

3. Protection: Put a clean, fresh gown or cutting square on the client.

4. Cleansing: Cleanse the client's skin in preparation for the massage service. Exfoliate if needed.

ACTIVITY

Different shops have different ways of doing things. Find out what your barber's shop procedures for maintaining towels are. Write down your answers in your portfolio:

1. At what point(s) in the day are towels washed?
2. What washing materials are used to wash the towels?
3. What wash cycle does the shop recommend?
4. How are the towels dried?
5. How are the towels stored and kept ready for use?

Preparing the client for shaving (Continued...)

STEP-BY-STEP: LATHERING

A rich lather is achieved by using a shaving brush or your fingers and should be applied quickly.

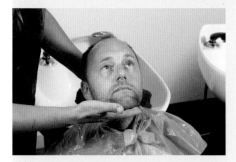

1 Put a clean, fresh gown and cutting square or disposable cape on the client.

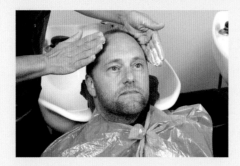

2 Cleanse the client's skin in preparation for the massage service. Exfoliate if needed.

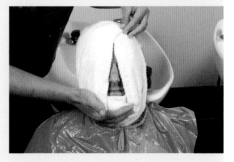

3 Apply a hot towel to the client's face to open up the pores in preparation for the massage. Remove the towel before it goes cold.

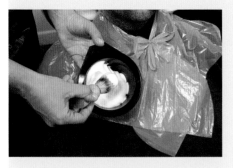

4 Build up a rich lather with the brush and apply in small circulatory movements all over the skin, but not extending beyond the area of beard hair. The movements should lift the beard. Apply brush strokes in a direction against the lie of the hair to produce the best results.

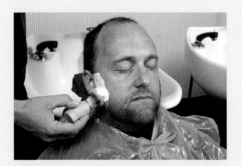

5 Apply the lather to one area of the beard at a time, not all over the beard area of the face. This prevents the skin from drying out.

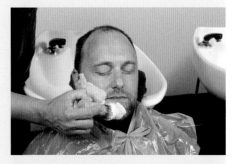

6 Take up to 3 or 4 minutes to apply and build up the lather; this will produce the best results for the shave. Inform the barber that the client is ready for his shave.

CourseMate video: Lathering

Telling the barber when the client is prepared

Prepare for the shave so that it fits in with the barber's other tasks and duties. There is no point starting any part of the process too soon because the benefits of what you are doing will be lost. Hot towels start cooling from the point that they are applied. If too much heat is lost prior to lathering, the follicles will start to close and the effectiveness of the shave will be lost. Similarly, the lather should be applied to a warm face to lubricate the surface of the skin and lift the facial hair. All of these are critical for the quality of the shave. Always make sure that you work closely with the barber and only start the preparation process when you have been told to. The moment the client is ready for shaving, let the barber know.

After the barber has completed the first time over and before the second

After the barber has used the **cut-throat razor** for the first time the skin can be treated with an alum block (potassium alum). There are several reasons for this:

◆ Alum helps to reduce redness and razor burn caused by the friction of shaving.

◆ It cleans the pores and the skin surface with its antiseptic properties.

◆ It stops any bleeding that may have occurred during the shave.

◆ As it is also an astringent it tightens the skin, providing better grip for the razor during the second shave.

The procedure is simple but very effective.

1. Wet your gloved hand with warm water and gently moisten the skin. The alum block should also be dipped into warm water (not hot).

2. In a gentle buffing motion run the block across the surface of the skin. Pay particular attention to red areas or bleeds by moving the alum block in small circular motions until you are satisfied that the alum has penetrated the skin.

3. Use the full surface of the block – ends for bleeds and redness, side for lip and broad side for main facial area.

It is important to not allow the block to dry out, so continuous wetting with water should be adhered to during the course of the procedure. Once this is finished, then the block should be dried and returned to its container or box. The barber will then complete the second time over. This will be working upwards against the natural growth to achieve a cleaner, closer shave.

HEALTH & SAFETY

Remember that for hygienic reasons and to reduce the risk of contamination, a new block should be used for each shave, with the used block being handed to the client at the end of the shave to take home.

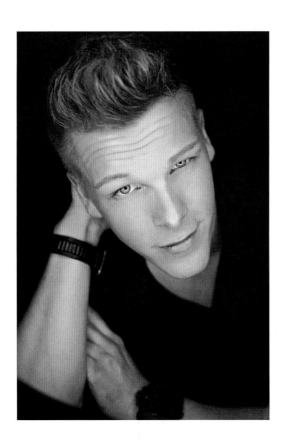

Completing the service

Removing lather and cooling the skin

The final stage of the shaving process is to cool the skin and close the hair follicles. Before this can happen, any remaining lather must be removed using a damp towel or sponge. Pat the face dry, taking care not to drag or pull the skin because the client's skin can still be quite sensitive.

Now apply a cool towel, which can be prepared by pre-soaking in a basin of cold water. Take the towel out of the basin and wring out the excess moisture. Apply in a similar way to hot towels, so that the nose is not covered. Leave for a few minutes and then remove the towels and place them in the towel bin.

Finally, complete the service by applying a little talcum powder (this dries the skin and prevents chapping), and the application of either an aftershave balm or lotion. An aftershave balm is more suitable to drier skin types because it helps to moisturize and lubricate the skin. A lotion can also be used; this is more zesty and suitable for normal to oily skin types.

TOP TIP

If you are applying lather by hand, wear close-fitting vinyl gloves. These will be more comfortable for the client and will stop your fingers slipping on the client's skin.

TOP TIP

Ask the client how cold they would like the cool towel to be. It can be a shock if the towel is very cold on an already warmed face.

Problems that you may encounter	
Problem	**Possible cause**
Client's skin is burned	Hot towels were not wrung out properly before application
	Hot towels too hot
Client develops rash after the shave	Tools not cleaned and sterilized properly
	Sterilizing chemicals not rinsed off equipment properly
	Client has in-growing hairs from shaving curly hair too closely
	Wrong shaving products applied
	Shaving products applied incorrectly
Uneven, patchy shave result	Hot towels not applied
	Hot towels allowed to cool down too much before shave is carried out
	Poor or uneven lather application
Client's skin sensitive after shave	Skin not allowed to cool properly
	Cool towels were not applied
	Shave was too close
	Poor or uneven lather application
	Talcum not applied
	Wrong shaving products applied
	Shaving products applied incorrectly

SUMMARY

Now you have finished this chapter you should have a clearer picture of all the essential aspects associated with assisting with shaping and trimming men's facial hair. In particular, you should now have a good understanding and be able to:

✓ prepare the client adequately for shaving services

✓ prepare the equipment safely and hygienically in readiness for shaving

✓ prepare the products associated with the service and apply them following the barber's explicit instructions

✓ work safely and hygienically at all times.

In addition, you will understand how these processes will enable you to work more efficiently and effectively in daily routines.

REVISION QUESTIONS

Q1. Copy and complete this sentence: The _____ block is used after the first time over to prevent razor burns.

Fill in the blank

Q2. Exfoliation removes the build-up of dead skin cells.

True or False

Q3. Which of the following are features of aftershave balms? (You may choose more than one answer.)

Cools the skin	☐	a
Exfoliates the skin	☐	b
Moisturizes the skin	☐	c
Prepares the skin for shaving	☐	d
Soothes the skin after shaving	☐	e
Should be applied with hot towels	☐	f

Q4. A badger brush is made of real badger hair.

True or False

Q5. Which is the finest quality real-hair shaving brush? (Choose one answer.)

Pure bristle	○	a
Best quality	○	b
Super quality	○	c
Nylon bristle	○	d

Health and safety legislation

This section provides you with an outline of the main health and safety regulations that affect hairdressers and barbers in their work.

Management of Health and Safety at Work Regulations 1999

The main regulation requires the employer to appoint competent personnel to conduct risk assessments for the health and safety of all staff working on the premises as well as visitors to the business premises. Staff must be adequately trained to take appropriate action, and eliminate or minimize any risks. Other regulations cover the necessity of setting up procedures for emergency situations and reviewing the risk assessment processes. In salons where five or more people are employed, there is the added obligation to set up a system for monitoring health surveillance, should the risk assessments identify a need.

The main requirements for management of health and safety are:

◆ identify any potential hazards

◆ assess the risks which could arise from these hazards and identify who is at risk

◆ eliminate or minimize the risks

◆ train staff to identify and control risks

◆ regularly review the assessment processes.

Workplace (Health, Safety and Welfare) Regulations 1992

These regulations supersede the Offices, Shops and Railway Premises Act 1963 (OSRPA) and cover the following workplace key points:

◆ maintenance of the workplace and the equipment in it

◆ sanitary and washing facilities

◆ drinking water supply

◆ resting, eating and changing facilities

◆ storage of clothing

◆ ventilation, temperature and lighting

◆ cleanliness

◆ glazing

◆ traffic routes

◆ workspace

Amendments and additions to this regulation provide new requirements for employers with particular attention for glazed areas such as windows and doors. Any transparent or translucent partitions must be made of safe materials and if they could cause injury to anyone they should be appropriately marked. Other amendments have particular rules for rest rooms and rest areas. These must include suitable alternative arrangements to protect non-smokers from the effects caused by tobacco smoke and suitable rest facilities for any person at work who is either pregnant or a nursing mother.

Health and Safety (First Aid) Regulations 1981

The Health and Safety (First Aid) Regulations 1981 require the employer to provide adequate and appropriate equipment, facilities and personnel to enable first aid to be given to their employees if they are injured or become ill at work.

The minimum first-aid provision on any work site is:

◆ a suitably stocked first aid box

◆ an appointed person to take charge of first aid arrangements.

It is also important to remember that accidents can happen at any time. First aid provision needs to be available at all times people are at work.

Personal Protective Equipment (PPE) at Work Regulations 1992

These relate to the requirement of employers to provide suitable and sufficient protective clothing and equipment for all employees to use. The PPE Regulations 1992 require managers to make an assessment of the processes and activities carried out at work and to identify where and when special items of clothing should be worn. In hairdressing environments, the potential hazards and dangers revolve around the task of providing hairdressing services – that is, in general, the application of hairdressing treatments and associated products.

Potentially hazardous substances used by hairdressers include:

◆ acidic solutions of varying strengths

◆ flammable liquids, often stored in pressurized containers

◆ caustic alkaline solutions of varying strengths

◆ vapours

◆ dyeing compounds.

There are also potentially hazardous items of equipment and their individual applications, such as:

◆ electrical appliances

◆ heated/heating instruments

◆ sharp cutting tools.

All these items require correct handling and safe usage procedures, and for several of them this includes the wearing of suitable items of protective equipment. Remember that not wearing appropriate gloves can lead to dermatitis.

Control of Substances Hazardous to Health (COSHH) Regulations 2003

Hairdressing employers are required by law to make an assessment of the exposure to all the substances used in their salon that could be potentially hazardous to themselves, their employees and salon visitors. The purpose of COSHH regulations is to make sure that people are working in the safest possible environment and conditions.

A substance is considered hazardous if it can cause harm to the body. It presents a risk if it is:

◆ in contact with the skin or eyes

◆ absorbed through the skin or via the eyes (either directly or from contact with contaminated surfaces or clothing)

◆ inhaled (breathed in from the atmosphere)

◆ ingested via contaminated food or finger-injected

◆ introduced to the body via cuts and abrasions.

Cosmetic Products (Safety) Regulations 2008

These regulations lay down the recommended volumes and percentage strengths of different hydrogen-based products. The strength will vary depending on whether it has been produced for professional or non-professional use. It is important that the manufacturer's guidance material and current legislation is checked when using or selling products.

Health and Safety (Information for Employees) Regulations 1989

This regulation requires the employer to make available to all employees notices, posters and leaflets either in the approved format or those actually published by the HSE.

Manual Handling Operations Regulations 1992

These regulations apply in all occupations where manual lifting occurs. They require employers to carry out a risk assessment of the work processes and activities that involve lifting, and provide the relevant training. The risk assessment should address detailed aspects of the following:

◆ any risk of injury

◆ the manual movement that is involved in the task

◆ the physical constraints the loads incur

- the work environmental constraints that are incurred

- the worker's individual capabilities

- steps and/or remedial action to take in order to minimize the risk.

Provision and Use of Work Equipment Regulations (PUWER) 1998

These regulations refer to the regular maintenance and monitoring of work equipment. Any equipment, new or second-hand, must be suitable for the purpose that it is intended. In addition to this, they require that anyone using this equipment must be adequately trained.

Electricity at Work Regulations 1989

These regulations require employers to maintain electrical equipment in a safe condition and to have it checked by a suitably qualified person. A written record of testing must be kept and made available for inspection. It is the employer's responsibility to provide training on handling and checking electrical equipment correctly. It is the employees' responsibility to report any known faulty equipment to their employer or supervisor. The following information must be kept:

- the electrician's/contractor's name, address, contact details

- an itemized list of salon electrical equipment along with serial numbers (for individual identification)

- the date of inspection

- the date of purchase/disposal.

Reporting of Injuries, Diseases and Dangerous Occurrences Regulations 1995 (RIDDOR)

Under these regulations there are certain diseases and groups of infections that, if sustained at work, are notifiable by law. So if any employees suffer a personal injury at work which results in one of the following, they must be reported to the appropriate authority:

- death

- major injuries, including: fractures (not fingers and toes), amputation, dislocation, loss of sight and other eye injuries

- more than 24 hours in hospital

- an incapacity to work for more than seven days.

People's rights and consumer legislation

Equality Act (2010)

This Act simplifies, strengthens and harmonizes the current legislation to provide a new discrimination law which protects individuals from unfair treatment and promotes a fair and more equal society.

It encompasses nine areas of legislation:

◆ Equal Pay Act 1970

◆ Sex Discrimination Act 1975

◆ Race Relations Act 1976

◆ Disability Discrimination Act 1995

◆ Employment Equality (Religion or Belief) Regulations 2003

◆ Employment Equality (Sexual Orientation) Regulations 2003

◆ Employment Equality (Age) Regulations 2006

◆ Equality Act 2006, Part 2

◆ Equality Act (Sexual Orientation) Regulations 2007

For more information visit: URL www.equalityhumanrights.com

Data Protection Act (1998)

Any organization that records information about staff or clients, whether on a card index system or a computer, must comply with the Data Protection Act. The law requires people to retain information securely about their customers. In salons, this means that information about clients must be kept confidential and handled with the utmost professional care. All staff working within the salon are responsible for maintaining this confidentiality at all times, even after working hours. You are not at liberty to discuss other peoples' circumstances with anyone.

Sale of Goods Act

Under the Sale of Goods Act, when a salon sells something to a customer they have an agreement or contract with them. A customer has legal rights if the goods they purchaed do not conform to contract (are faulty). The Act says that to conform to contract goods should:

1. **Match their description:** by law everything that is said about the product must not be misleading – whether this is said by a sales assistant, or written on the packaging, in-store, on advertising materials or in a catalogue.

2. **Be of satisfactory quality:** this quality of goods includes:
    - appearance and finish
    - freedom from minor defects (such as marks or holes)
    - safe to use
    - in good working order
    - durability.

3. **Be fit for purpose:** if a customer says – or when it should be obvious to the retailer – that an item is wanted for a particular purpose, even if it is a purpose the item is not usually supplied for, and the retailer agrees the item is suitable, or does not say it is not fit for that purpose, then it has to be reasonably fit. If there is disagreement with the customer about a particular purpose, the salon should make this clear, perhaps on the sales receipt, to protect the business against future claims.

Trades Descriptions Act 1968 / 1972

Products must not be falsely or misleadingly described in relation to their quality, fitness, price or purpose, by advertisements, orally, displays or descriptions. And since 1972 it has also been a requirement to label a product clearly, so that the buyer can see where the product was made.

Briefly, a retailer cannot:

◆   mislead consumers by making false statements about products

◆   offer sale products at half price unless they have been offered at the actual price for a reasonable period.

The Consumer Protection Act (1987)

This Act follows European laws to protect the buyer in the following areas:

◆   **Product liability:** a customer may claim compensation for a product that doesn't reach general standards of safety

◆   **General safety requirements:** it is a criminal offence to sell goods that are unsafe; traders that breach this conduct may face fines or even imprisonment

◆   **Misleading prices:** misleading consumers with wrongly displayed prices is also an offence.

The Act is designed to help safeguard the consumer from products that do not reach reasonable levels of safety. Your salon will take adequate precautions in procuring, using and supplying reputable products and maintaining them so that they remain in good condition.

Revision section answer key

Chapter One	Answers		Chapter Two	Answers
Q1	Blow-dry		Q1	Infestation
Q2	True		Q2	True
Q3	C E		Q3	4 5
Q4	Trichologist		Q4	False
Q5	True		Q5	C

Chapter Three	Answers		Chapter Four	Answers
Q1	Harm		Q1	Client
Q2	True		Q2	True
Q3	1 3 6		Q3	1 2 5 6
Q4	True		Q4	True
Q5	D		Q5	4

Chapter Five	Answers		Chapter Six	Answers
Q1	Confidential		Q1	Removing
Q2	True		Q2	False
Q3	4 5		Q3	1 4
Q4	True		Q4	False
Q5	A		Q5	C

Chapter Seven	Answers		Chapter Eight	Answers
Q1	Sterilized		Q1	Traction
Q2	True		Q2	True
Q3	1 5		Q3	1 3
Q4	True		Q4	True
Q5	B		Q5	C

Chapter Nine	Answers		Chapter Ten	Answers
Q1	Dissolve		Q1	Fade
Q2	False		Q2	True
Q3	2 3 4 5		Q3	2 3
Q4	True		Q4	True
Q5	B		Q5	A

Chapter Eleven	Answers		Chapter Twelve	Answers
Q1	Fix		Q1	Alum
Q2	True		Q2	True
Q3	1 2 3		Q3	1 3 5
Q4	True		Q4	True
Q5	C		Q5	C

Useful addresses and websites

Business

Arbitration, Conciliation and Advisory Service (ACAS)
ACAS National (Head Office)
Euston Tower
286 Euston Road
London
NW1 3JJ
Tel: 08457 38 37 36
URL **www.acas.org.uk**
Call the Helpline on 08457 47 47 47
Monday to Friday 8am–8pm; Saturday 9am–1pm

Hairdressing Employers Association (HEA)
10 Coldbath Square
London
EC1R 5HL
Tel: 020 7833 0633

Training and Education

Hairdressing and Beauty Industry Authority (Habia)
Oxford House
Sixth Avenue
Sky Business Park
Robin Hood Airport
Doncaster
DN9 3GG
Tel: 0845 2 306080
Fax: 01302 774949
URL **www.habia.org**

Association of Colleges (AOC)
2–5 Stedham Place
London
WC1A 1HU
Tel: 020 7034 9900
Fax: 020 7034 9950

City and Guilds (C&G)
1 Giltspur Street
London
EC1A 9DD
Tel: 020 7294 2800
URL **www.city-and-guilds.co.uk**

The Institute of Trichologists
107 Trinity Road
Upper Tooting
London
SW17 7SQ
Tel: 0845 604 4657
URL **www.trichologists.org.uk**

Vocational Training Charitable Trust (VTCT)
Prysmian House
Dew Lane
Eastleigh
Hampshire
SO50 9PX
Tel: +44 (0) 2380 684 500
Fax: 02380 651493
URL **www.vtct.org.uk**

ITEC
2nd floor, Chiswick Gate
598-608 Chiswick High Road
London
W4 5RT
Tel: +44 (0)20 8994 4141
URL **http://www.itecworld.co.uk/**

World Federation of Hairdressing and Beauty Schools
PO Box 367
Coulsdon
Surrey
CR5 2TP
Tel: 01737 551355

Hairdressing Course Information
URL **www.learnhairdressing.net**
URL **www.learnabouthair.com**

Publications / Fashion Forecasting

Hairdressers Journal International (HJ)
Quadrant House
The Quadrant, Sutton
Surrey
SM2 5AS
Tel: 020 8652 3500
URL **www.hji.co.uk**

Creative Head
21 The Timberyard
Drysdale Street
London,
N1 6ND
Tel: 020 7324 7540
Fax: 020 7739 7789
URL **www.creativeheadmag.com**

Runway Magazine
URL **www.runwaybeauty.com**

Black Beauty and Hair
Culvert House
Culvert Road
London
SW11
Tel: 020 7720 2108
URL **www.blackbeautyandhair.com**

Trade Associations

British Association of Beauty Therapy and Cosmetology Limited (BABTAC)
BABTAC Ltd,
Ambrose House
Meteor Court, Barnett Way
Barnwood
Gloucester
GL4 3GG
URL **www.babtac.com**

Cosmetic, Toiletry and Perfumery Association (CTPA)
Josaron House
5–7 John Princes Street
London
W1G 0JN
Tel: 020 7491 8891
URL **www.ctpa.org.uk**
URL **www.thefactsabout.co.uk**

Fellowship for British Hairdressing
Bloxham Mill
Barford Road
Bloxham
Banbury
Oxon.
Tel: 01295 724579
URL **www.fellowshiphair.com/**

Freelance Hair and Beauty Federation
FHBF Head Office
The Business Centre
Kimpton Road
Luton
Beds.
LU2 0LB
URL **www.fhbf.org.uk**

The Hairdressing and Beauty Suppliers Association
Greenleaf House
128 Darkes Lane
Potters Bar
Hertfordshire
EN6 1AE
Tel: 01707 649499
Fax: 01707
URL **www.hbsa.uk.com**

The Hairdressing Council (HC)
30 Sydenham Road
Croydon
CR0 2EF
Tel: 020 8771 6205
URL **www.haircouncil.org.uk**

Health and Beauty Employers Federation (part of the Federation of Holistic Therapists)
18 Shakespeare Business Centre
Hathaway Close
Eastleigh
Hampshire
SO50 4SR
URL **www.fht.org.uk**

Incorporated Guild of Hairdressers, Wigmakers and Perfumers
Langdale Road
Barnsley
South Yorkshire
S71 1AQ
Tel: 01226 786 555
Fax: 01226 731 814

National Hairdressers' Federation (NHF)
One Abbey Court
Fraser Road
Priory Business Park
Bedford
MK44 3WH
Tel: 01234 831965 or 0845 345 6500
URL **www.the-nhf.org**

Legal and Regulatory

Health and Safety Executive
Publications
PO Box 1999
Sudbury
Suffolk
CO10 6FS
(HSE) Infoline
Tel: 0845 345 0055
URL **www.hse.gov.uk**

Equality and Human Rights Commission
Equality Advisory Support Service
Tel: 0808 800 0082
URL **http://www.equalityhumanrights.com**

Union of Shop, Distributive and Allied Workers (USDAW)
188 Wilmslow Road
Fallowfield
Manchester
M14 6LJ
Tel: 0161 224 2804 / 249 2400

Glossary

Accident book a record of accidents within the workplace required by health and safety law

Alpha keratin the state the hair is in before stretching and setting into a new shape

Ammonium thioglycolate an alkaline substance in perm lotions that reacts with the disulphide bonds

Anti-oxidant conditioner stops the oxidation process of chemical services

Antiseptics reduces the growth of micro-organisms that cause disease

Appointment system the efficient way of organizing salon work

Appraisal a process of reviewing work performance over a period of time

Bacteria a tiny organism that can only be seen under a microscope

Barrier cream a cream that protects the skin against harmful moisture or infection

Beta keratin the state the hair is in after it has been stretched and set into a new shape

Body language non-verbal communication provided by gestures, expressions and mannerisms

Body odour (BO) the result of poor personal hygiene and lack of regular washing

Cane rows see **Cornrows**

Client care maintaining goodwill while developing regular, repeated business

Cold-fusion hair extensions a system of connecting hair extensions by using adhesives and adhesive strips

Confidentiality the professional way of handling client information

Congo plait see **French plait**

Cornrows (also known as cane rows) a term used to describe an effect created by multiple rows of plaits that follow the contour of the head

Cortex the inner part of the hair where most chemical processes take place

COSHH an abbreviation for Control of Substances Hazardous to Health; these are health and safety regulations affecting you in your work

Cross-infection the transmission of infectious microorganisms from one person to another

Cross-infestation the transmission of animal parasites from one person to another

Cuticle the outer protective layer of the hair resembling overlapping tiles on a roof

Dermatitis an occupational disease that affects the skin causing an itching sensation accompanied by reddening and dry cracked areas

Disinfection does not kill all organisms like sterilization, but slows down the rate of growth of bacteria

Disulphide bonds the chemical bonds within the hair that are rearranged during perming and neutralizing

Effective communication professional communication that is not ambiguous, providing clear instruction or information

Effleurage a light stroking movement applied with either the fingers or the palms of the hands

Emulsify a way of mixing the colour with water in order to remove it from the hair

Exfoliate to scrub skin with a gritty substance to remove the dead cells of the surface layer

French plait (also known as Congo plait/Guinea plait) a three-strand plait that starts, centrally, near the front hairline and continues closely to the scalp to the nape and continues as a freely hanging plait beyond

Friction a firm, vigorous rubbing massage technique made by the fingertips, used during shampooing

Goodwill the reputation of a business formed by the people who work for it

Guinea plait see **French plait**

Hair trap a flexible nylon or plastic plug that helps to stop hair from entering the drain

Halitosis bad breath

Hazard something with potential to cause harm

Hot-bonded hair extensions a system of connecting hair extensions by using resin or hard plastics

Humidity the moisture level in the air

Hydrophilic water loving

Hydrophobic water repelling

Legislation laws created by parliament

Medulla the central part of the hair that is only found in coarser hair types

Melanin the naturally occurring pigments formed within the skin and hair

Moisturizing balms cooling, soothing and moisture replenishing lotions applied after shaving to counteract the abrasive effects of the process

Neutralizer a chemical compound which is used to both balance and fix hair that has been previously permed

Pathogen something that can cause disease, e.g. a bacterium or a virus

Personal development plan an ongoing action plan for self-improvement that defines personal objectives or targets, set over a period of time (often reviewed during appraisal)

Petrissage a kneading movement of the skin that lifts and compresses underlying structures of the skin, often used when applying conditioner

pH balance the natural acid mantle of skin and hair at pH5.5

pH level a measurement of a solution that denotes whether it is alkaline (pH 8-14), or acid (pH 6-1)

Pigment a granular form of colouration that can be natural or artificial

Practice block a modelling head with longer hair that can be attached to a work surface for practising techniques

Removal solution a chemical formulated to dissolve the adhesive connecting the hair extension to the hair in cold-fusion systems

Removal tool a metal pair of pliers used for breaking the bond connecting the hair extension to the hair in hot-bonded systems

Revenue stream a source of income that comes into a business, e.g. retail sales, sales of services, sales of treatments

Risk assessment the process of assessing hazards within the workplace

Risk the likelihood of a hazard's potential being realized

Rotary a quicker and firmer circulatory movement used in shampooing

Senegalese twists a twisting technique that resembles the plaited effect created by cornrows

Sharps the name given to sharp items, e.g. razor blades

Sharps box a designated sealed container used for the safe disposal of sharp items, e.g. used razor blades

Sterilization the complete eradication of living organisms

Stock rotation when shelves are re-stocked the newer product is put at the back and the older stock is brought to the front; to be sold first

Surface conditioner a light conditioner that works on the outside of the hair to smooth and fill areas of damaged, missing or worn cuticle until the next shampoo

Traction alopecia a condition that is caused by the excessive pulling of hair at the root, it is often associated with longer hair worn in plaits, twists, hair-ups and extensions

Virgin hair a hairdressing term describing hair that has never been coloured

Index

Notes